Thinking About Health
A Student Resource Manual

for

Donatelle and Davis

Access to Health
Sixth Edition

Prepared by

Lynne Blesz Vestal

Allyn and Bacon
Boston London Toronto Sydney Tokyo Singapore

A Pearson Education Company
160 Gould Street
Needham Heights, Massachusetts 02494-2130

Internet: www.abacon.com

ISBN 0-205-30505-9

Printed in the United States of America

10 9 8 7 6 5 4 3 2 1   03 02 01 00 99

TABLE OF CONTENTS

Preface to the Student v

1 Promoting Healthy Behavior Change 1

2 Psychosocial Health:
Being Mentally, Emotionally, Socially, and Spiritually Well 15

3 Managing Stress:
Coping with Life's Challenges 25

4 Intentional and Unintentional Injuries:
Staying Safe in a Violent World 35

5 Communicating Effectively:
A Key to Interpersonal Health 43

6 Healthy Relationships:
Friends, Family, and Significant Others 51

7 Sexuality:
Defining Your Sexual Behavior 61

8 Birth Control, Pregnancy, and Childbirth:
Managing Your Fertility 71

9 Addictions and Addictive Behavior:
Threats to Wellness 83

10 Pharmaceutical Drugs:
Safe and Responsible Use 91

11 Drinking Responsibly:
A Lifestyle Challenge 101

12 Tobacco and Caffeine:
Legal Addictions 111

13 Illicit Drugs:
Use, Misuse, and Abuse 121

14 Nutrition:
Eating for Optimum Health 129

15 Managing Your Weight:
Finding a Healthy Balance 141

16 Personal Fitness:
Improving Your Health Through Exercise 149

17 Cardiovascular Disease:
Helping The Beat Go On....159

18 Cancer:
Reducing Your Risks....167

19 Infectious Diseases and Sexually Transmitted Infections:
Reducing Risks and Increasing Responsibilities....173

20 Noninfectious Conditions:
The Modern Maladies....183

21 Healthy Aging:
A Lifelong Process....191

22 Dying and Death:
The Final Transition....199

23 Environmental Health:
Thinking Globally, Acting Locally....207

24 Consumerism:
Selecting Health-Care Products and Services....215

PREFACE TO THE STUDENT

This Study Guide was designed to facilitate your understanding of health. By working on each corresponding chapter in your textbook, you will become an active participant in the learning process. Active participation involves more than just attending the lectures and reading the textbook--it means that you ask questions, hypothesize, are skeptical of some reported results, doubt some of the research findings, discover how concepts of health apply specifically to your life, and develop new questions to ask until you realize that you have more questions than answers.

Engage yourself in this learning process! When you do, you will become a critical thinker of health. When using critical thinking, you should question every fact and challenge every assumption, always asking yourself, "Do I agree with what the author is saying?" Another aspect of critical thinking is applying concepts of health to your own life, always asking yourself, "How does this concept apply to me?"

Each chapter of this study guide corresponds with the chapters of *Access to Health, 6e*, with each following a very basic organizational structure. Each chapter includes:

Chapter Overview
The chapter overview serves as a useful comprehensive summary in your reading of the textbook.

Learning Objectives
Before you read each chapter, scan the objectives to see what you are going to read. After reading each chapter and working on the questions in the student resource manual, you should be meet each of the objectives.

Key Terms
The key terms provide a helpful preview of key terms to be addressed in the textbook. Writing a brief definition of each key term in your own words will help you remember the important concepts.

Short Answers
This set of exercises includes items that are factual or conceptual in nature.

Critical Thinking Exercises
This set of exercises requires you to apply your knowledge from the text to real-life or hypothetical situations.

Critical Thinking Activity
Each chapter includes a critical thinking activity. The purpose of the activity is to facilitate critical thinking, and to help you learn to become a critical evaluator of health.

Using Your *Access to Health* Interactive Companion

Another valuable resource for you is the Interactive Companion CD-ROM that accompanies your main text. Using chapter highlights as the organizing structure of the CD-ROM, the IC encourages you to apply what you have learned by presenting you with hundreds of links to audio and video clips, web sites, activities, and practice tests. These links are annotated with brief descriptions that help you understand the value and purpose of each media asset in the context of the chapter. The IC guides you through your studies and helps you reach beyond the covers of the printed text. Here are some suggestions for how the Interactive Companion might help you better understand health concepts and prepare for your classroom assignments and discussions:

Concept Clarification:

- Video and audio clips can bring concepts to life by acting as living examples of topics you read about in your text
- Use the Web links on the CD-ROM as the basis for further investigation into the subjects discussed in the book . Some of the links will take you to sites for ongoing research into issues discussed in the book (i.e. the Human Genome Project, the Framingham Heart Study), allowing you the opportunity for immediate updates on the status of the findings.

Critical Thinking

At various points, you'll have the opportunity to respond to questions that pry into the meaning of the readings and explore further possibilities and considerations. Depending on your university's capabilities, you may have the opportunity to share your thoughts online with classmates and your instructor, creating an interactive environment guaranteed to stimulate even more discussion on the topics.

Self-Assessment

Complete activities designed to explore your personal attitudes and see how you score. Scoring and feedback is provided immediately.

Practice Tests

Each chapter contains an electronic practice test that helps you prepare for quizzes and tests by testing your current knowledge. After completing each test, you can determine your score with the click of a button. You can use the practice tests in a couple of ways:

- Complete each test after reading the chapter to test your retention level and assess your knowledge. This method will help you determine your level of preparedness for testing in class.
- Complete the practice test before reading the chapter to assess your level of knowledge prior to instruction and reading. Once you've completed the readings and in-class discussion on the subject matter is complete, you might want to take the test again to see if you've improved your knowledge level on the subject.

Used to its fullest, the Interactive Companion CD-ROM can become your best study tool!

CHAPTER 1
PROMOTING HEALTHY BEHAVIOR CHANGE

Chapter Overview

Today, the terms *health* and *wellness* are often used interchangeably to mean the dynamic, ever-changing process of trying to achieve one's individual potential in each of several interrelated dimensions: physical, intellectual, social, emotional, environmental, and spiritual health. This definition of health proposes a positive view that focuses on our individual attempts to achieve optimum well-being within a realistic framework of our individual potential. Health can be described on a continuum from premature death to optimal well-being. Many people believe in taking a holistic approach to wellness, with an emphasis on the integration of the mind, body, and spirit.

The term *health promotion* describes the educational, organizational, procedural, environmental, social, and financial supports that help individuals and groups reduce negative health behaviors and promote positive change. Health promotion programs identify healthy people who are at risk for disease and attempt to motivate them to improve their health status. The focus of prevention is on taking positive actions now to avoid becoming sick later. Although there are three major types of prevention—primary, secondary, and tertiary—the emphasis of prevention today is on the role of prevention specialists and prevention programs.

There are key differences in health status between men and women. For instance, although women have longer lifespans than do men, they don't necessarily have a better quality of life. The National Institutes of Health (NIH) established the Office of Research on Women's Health (ORWH) in 1990 to oversee the representation of women in National Institutes of Health (NIH) studies, following a concern about uneven numbers of women included in clinical trial research by the NIH. In addition, the NIH launched the Women's Health Initiative (WHI), a study focusing on the leading causes of death and disease in postmenopausal women. And, the NIH has stated that equal amounts of money and time must be spent on men's and women's health research.

Risks for the leading causes of death in the United States have been reduced significantly by practicing specific lifestyle patterns, such as regular exercise and stress management.

Prochaska and DiClemente's Stages of Change Model helps explain why people succeed or fail in their attempts to change behavior. Predisposing factors, enabling factors, and reinforcing factors influence behavior and behavioral-change decisions. In addition, our beliefs and attitudes will significantly affect what we do. The health belief model and the theory of reasoned action are useful models for explaining why people behave in a particular way. According to the health belief model, when perceived severity, perceived susceptibility, and cues to action support a belief, change is likely to occur. The theory of reasoned action explains that behaviors result from our intentions to carry out a behavior. The more consistent and powerful your attitudes about an action are and the more you are influenced by others to take that action, the greater will be your stated intention to do so. In addition, significant others influence our health behaviors, both positively and negatively.

Once you have analyzed influences on your current behavior and all the factors that may influence the desired behavior change, you must decide which technique for behavior change will work best for you. Techniques include shaping, visualization, modeling, situational inducement, reinforcement, and changing self-talk.

One method of modifying your behavior is to conduct a self-assessment of the antecedents and consequences of a situation to help you look at the circumstances in which your behavior occurs, and then analyze its components. Then, when you decide to change a behavior, you will be faced with choices. By developing your decision-making skills, you increase your chances of making the choice you really want to make. Finally, set behavior-change goals that are realistic for you.

Learning Objectives

1. Define health and wellness, and explain the interconnected roles of the physical, social, mental, emotional, environmental, and spiritual dimensions of health.

2. Discuss the importance of health promotion and disease prevention and differentiate among the major prevention types.

3. Discuss the health status of Americans, the factors that contribute to health, and the importance of Healthy People 2000, Healthy People 2010, and the AHCPR guidelines in establishing national goals for promoting health and preventing premature death and disability.

4. Provide a rationale for focusing on current risk behaviors as a means of influencing a current and future health status.

5. Evaluate the role of gender in health status, health research, and health training.

6. Identify the leading causes of death and the lifestyle patterns associated with the reduction of risks.

7. Examine how predisposing factors, beliefs, attitudes, and significant others affect your behavior changes.

8. Survey behavior change techniques, and learn how to apply them to personal situations.

9. Apply decision-making techniques to behavior changes.

Key Terms

Fill in a brief definition to help you remember these terms.

health ______________________________

mortality ______________________________

morbidity ______________________________

wellness ______________________________

health promotion ______________________________

disease prevention ______________________________

primary prevention ______________________________

secondary prevention ______________________________

tertiary prevention ______________________________

belief ______________________________

attitude ______________________________

health belief model ______________________________

theory of reasoned action ____

shaping ____

imagined rehearsal ____

modeling ____

situational inducement ____

positive reinforcement ____

Activities of Daily Living (ADL)____

Objectives of the Nation____

AHCPR Guidelines____

risk behaviors____

Certified Health Education Specialists____

Women's Health Initiative____

Short Answers

1. Define health.

2. What types of support do health promotion programs use to help people change negative health behaviors?

3. Identify and define one level of disease prevention.

4. What key behaviors are believed to help people live longer?

5. Identify three factors that influence behavior-change decisions and provide an example of each.

6. Distinguish between belief and attitude.

7. According to the Health Belief Model (HBM), what factors must support a belief in order for change to be likely to occur?

8. Define situational inducement and provide an example of how a positive situational inducement could improve behavior change.

9. Identify and provide examples of five types of positive reinforcers.

10. List reasons for why people fail in their efforts to change a given behavior.

Critical Thinking Exercises

1. Health is multidimensional. Using the following scenario, apply the dimensions of health to Heidi's different components of health: Heidi is a 34-year-old married female with two children. She is a partner in a law firm specializing in environmental law and works approximately 70 hours per week. She has a medium frame and is physically fit. Heidi is extremely competitive, both in her personal life and her work life. She competes in running marathons five times a year and publishes several law articles annually. She adapts well to a variety of social situations but tends not to always interact well with co-workers, as she has a high need for control. She describes herself as private and rarely expresses her feelings, except in an aggressive manner at work. She is also quite active in a volunteer program that educates the public on environmental issues. She has recently become involved in a church to which her husband already belongs.

____

____

____

____

____

2. According to the Global Burden of Disease, a projection for ranking major threats to health, unipolar major depression is projected as becoming the leading cause of disease burden (in female and developing countries). What factors do you think contribute to this health threat? What can be done to diminish this growing problem?

____

____

____

____

____

3. According to James Prochaska and Carlos DiClimente, we must go through a series of "stages" to ready ourselves for eventual change. Identify a behavior you have already changed and the stages you went through to prepare yourself for that change.

____

____

____

____

____

4. Identify at least 5 health promotion efforts available to you where you live. How does each program enhance the likelihood that, once a person decides to change a behavior, conditions are optimal for his or her success?

5. Identify a behavior you need to change. What stage of change are you in? What strategies would help you change?

6. Pedro is a sophomore in college. He smokes two packs of cigarettes a day. He started smoking when he was fifteen. When his roommate warned him of the hazards of smoking, Pedro replied, "I'm going to die somehow, so I might as well enjoy myself." Using the health belief model as a framework for discussion, explain what factors Pedro must consider before he will stop smoking.

7. Identify ways in which your family, friends, and other people have influenced your health behaviors.

8. Suppose you are a physical fitness expert. Your client, Yolanda, has not exercised for years. She explains that she went to her doctor for a physical exam and the doctor encouraged her to become physically fit. Yolanda decided she wants to be able to jog four miles daily. Develop a plan of action that uses a series of incremental steps to get Yolanda to her goal, and include guidelines for shaping her behavior.

9. Explain how the technique of visualization, or imagined rehearsal, could help someone who wants to be more assertive at work.

10. Explain the basic premise of rational-emotive therapy. Provide a statement that contains irrational self-talk and replace that statement with a positive, rational one.

____

____

____

____

____

Critical Thinking Activity: A Self-Assessment

Identify one health behavior that you would like to change. Conduct your own self-assessment by monitoring the antecedents and consequences of your behavior. Use the following worksheet to help you in your assessment.

SELF-ASSESSMENT

I choose to change the following health behavior:

Antecedents

(List the setting events for your behavior that cue or stimulate you to act in certain ways, such as physical events, thoughts, emotions, inner self-talk, or other people.)

Behavior

(Identify the behavior.)

Consequences

(List the results of your behavior that affect whether you will repeat it or not.)

Questions for the Critical Thinker

Analyze the health behavior that you want to change by noting the following characteristics:

1. Frequency (How often am I engaging in this behavior? All of the time or only once in awhile?)

2. Duration (Have I been engaging in this behavior for a long time? How long?)

3. Seriousness (What are the consequences of my behavior for me? For others?)

4. Basis for Problem Behavior (Is my behavior based on facts or my own perceptions of the facts?)

5. Antecedents. (What kind of situations trigger the behavior? Do some settings or people bring out the behavior more so than others? Why am I engaging in this behavior?)

Next, set goals that are realistic and workable for you. The following questions will give you valuable insights into your behaviors:

1. What is it I want?

2. Which change is of greatest priority at this time?

3. Why is this important to me?

4. What are the potential positive outcomes?

5. What health-promoting programs and services are available to help me get started?

6. Are there family or friends whose help I can enlist?

Language Enrichment Glossary

In addition to the words in the Key Terms list at the end of the chapter, students listed the following words as difficult to understand. Use the chapter Key Terms list, this list, your dictionary, and teachers and friends to learn the meaning of words you do not understand.

abnormal:	unusual
acknowledge:	recognize, accept
adherence to:	obedience to
antecedents:	events occurring before
anticipate:	expect
appraisal:	assessment
attributes:	characteristics
berate:	criticize
buffeted:	pushed back and forth roughly
catastrophic:	disastrous
chronic:	periodic, persistent, long-lasting
clinical trial:	research tests
cliches:	common sayings
cliques:	exclusive social groups
coaxed:	persuaded
cognitive procedures:	thought processes
complex:	complicated
conclude:	assume
condiments:	things to flavor food
congratulate:	compliment
consistent:	in agreement with
constitute:	are made up of
conveyed:	carried or taught
coping:	managing
couldn't care less:	don't care
criteria:	guidelines
criticism:	negative judgments

cues:	reminders
deficient:	missing something
deserted:	left
determinant:	cause
devastated:	destroyed in large numbers
deviations:	moving away from
devising:	developing
dimension:	part
dimensions:	areas
dread:	anticipate with bad feelings
dwell on:	think about often
dynamic:	changing
dysfunctional:	not working well
embellishments:	unneeded extra things
enabling:	making possible
enhance:	increase
entity:	something
external trappings:	decorations
extrapolate:	make assumptions from
factors:	causes
feeling component:	emotions
flung:	tossed
foolproof:	error-free
foster:	encourage
fundamental grounding:	basic teaching
gender:	male or female
generalities:	broad statements
genetic predispositions:	inherited tendencies
genetic:	inherited through the genes
getting down and dirty:	saying bad things about someone
gift of gab:	ability to talk well
gorging yourself:	eating too much
gossiping:	talking about someone
holistic:	looking at the whole
hygiene:	clean health practices
idle chatter:	casual talk
immunity:	protected from something
immunized:	vaccinated
indicators:	measurements
insignificant:	not important
instilled:	taught
interactions:	communication between people
irrational:	not logical
landmark:	point used as a basis for comparison
life expectancy:	number of years lived
life span:	length of life
lifestyle patterns:	ways of living
lousy:	bad
maintain currency:	stay up-to-date
monetary:	money

mounting:	increasing
nonjudgmental:	not critical
norms:	customs
optimal:	maximum
ostracism:	isolation
overkill:	too much
oversee:	supervise
perspective:	outlook
physiological:	physical
predisposing:	creating a tendency toward
preoccupied:	distracted by
prerequisite:	initial requirement
primary:	most important
priority areas:	things of importance
quality time:	well-used time
rational:	logical, sensible
reinforcing:	encouraging
sanitize:	clean
sauteed:	lightly fried
self-efficacy:	personal competence
sensory acuity:	sharpness of the senses
significant others:	close relationships
solely:	only
sound:	strong
spectrum:	range
stick to your limit:	avoid going beyond your maximum
structured to exert:	designed to apply
subtly:	not obviously
susceptibility:	easy to become ill
trigger:	cause, stimulate
unconditional trust:	complete trust
unfit:	poor condition
variables:	various things
verbalize:	say
visualize:	imagine
vital statistic:	information about people
zeal:	eagerness
zealot:	extreme enthusiast

CHAPTER 2
PSYCHOSOCIAL HEALTH:
BEING MENTALLY, EMOTIONALLY, SOCIALLY AND SPIRITUALLY WELL

Chapter Overview

Psychosocial health consists of mental, emotional, social, and spiritual dimensions of health. Mental health refers to the "thinking" part of psychosocial wellness. It includes such intellectual processes as the ability to reason, remember, interpret, evaluate, and solve problems. Emotional health involves the "feeling," or subjective, side of psychosocial health. Emotions are intensified feelings or complex patterns of feelings that we experience every minute of the day. Emotions include loving, caring, hating, hurt, despair, release, joy, anxiety, fear, frustration, and anger. Social health is the part of psychosocial health dealing with our interactions with others and our ability to adapt to social situations. Our social health is tied to strong social bonds and key social supports. Spiritual health refers to a belief in some unifying force that gives a sense of purpose or meaning to our lives or a sense of belonging to a greater scheme of existence.

Our psychosocial health depends upon how we perceive our life experiences. While some experiences are under our control, others are not. Many external factors influence psychosocial health, including the family and the greater environment, as well as internal factors, such as our hereditary traits, physical health status, personality, and maturity.

Your well-being is largely determined by your ability to respond to life's challenges and can be defined by your level of self-fulfillment. Attaining self-fulfillment is a lifelong process that involves building self-esteem, understanding and controlling emotions, and learning to solve problems and make decisions. The relationships we had with our parents and family when we were children have much to do with our self-esteem. Self-esteem can be enhanced through finding a support group, completing required tasks, forming realistic expectations, taking time for you, maintaining physical health, and examining problems and seeking help. Some researchers believe that negative emotions can make people physically sick and positive emotions can boost people's immune systems. Although there is a large body of evidence pointing to at least a minor association between emotions and physical health, there is still no definitive proof of such a relationship.

Common psychosocial problems include depression, obsessive-compulsive disorders, anxiety disorders (including phobias, panic attacks, and post-traumatic stress syndrome), seasonal affective disorder, and schizophrenia. Suicide is often a result of negative psychosocial reactions to life. Among the risk factors for suicide are a family history of suicide, previous suicide attempts, excessive drug and alcohol use, prolonged depression, financial difficulties, serious illness in the suicide contemplator or in his or her loved ones, and loss of a loved one through death or rejection. Most people who commit suicide signal their intentions. There are a number of actions to take if someone threatens suicide or displays warning signs.

The number of Americans who are turning to mental health professionals for help with psychosocial problems is increasing, most likely due to a breakdown in support systems, high expectations of the individual by society, and dysfunctional families.

Learning Objectives

1. Define psychosocial health in terms of mental, emotional, social, and spiritual components, and identify the basic elements shared by psychosocially healthy people.

2. Identify the internal and external factors influencing psychosocial health and consider how each may have affected you.

3. Discuss the positive steps you can take to enhance your psychosocial health.

4. Identify and describe common psychosocial problems of young adulthood and explain their causes and available treatments.

5. Discuss the mind/body connection in determining overall health status.

6. Illustrate the warning signs of suicide and what actions can be taken to help a suicidal individual.

7. Evaluate the role gender plays in diagnoses of mental health and the risks for selected mental health problems.

8. Identify the different types of mental health professionals and strategies for selecting a good therapist.

Key Terms

Fill in a brief definition to help you remember these terms.

psychosocial health ______________________________

mental health ______________________________

emotional health ______________________________

emotions ______________________________

social bonds ______________________________

social supports ______________________________

prejudice ______________________________

dysfunctional families ______________________________

self-efficacy ______________________________

personal control ______________________________

learned helplessness ______________________________

self-esteem ______________________________

endogenous depression ______________________________

exogenous depression ______________________________

obsessive-compulsive disorder ______________________________

anxiety disorders ______________________________

phobia ______________________________

panic attack ____

seasonal affective disorder (SAD) ______________________________

schizophrenia ____

psychiatrist ____

psychoanalyst ____

psychologist ____

social worker ____

counselor ____

Short Answers

1. Identify four basic types of emotions.

2. What two factors of social health are particularly important?

3. What does it mean to be spiritually healthy?

4. What role does self-efficacy play in enhancing our psychosocial health?

5. List six ways to boost your self-esteem.

6. Distinguish between endogenous and exogenous depression.

7. Distinguish between an obsession and a compulsion.

8. Name three major types of anxiety disorders.

9. What are risk factors for seasonal affective disorder?

10. What are some ways to build your self-esteem?

Critical Thinking Exercises

1. As a college residence hall director, Paul is concerned about the psychosocial health of the residents. You are the dean of the college's psychology department. Paul asks you to list the basic elements shared by psychologically healthy people. What do you tell him?

____

____

____

____

____

2. Suppose that your friend has had insomnia for the past month. She is about to turn to over-the-counter sleeping pills or tranquilizers to get some sleep. What methods can you suggest that would be less harmful?

____

____

____

____

____

3. Your friend tells you that he has been diagnosed with depression. He shares with you that he will be treated with a combination of cognitive therapy and interpersonal therapy. How are these two types of therapy similar? How do they differ?

____

____

____

____

____

4. Suppose you observe that your friend has withdrawn from her family and friends and from activities she once enjoyed. She has lost interest in classes and has been depressed following the breakup of a long relationship. She confides to you that she "can't take it" and says that she "might as well end it all." You are concerned that she might attempt suicide. What actions can you take?

____

____

____

____

____

5. Yuri, your business partner, is reluctant to seek professional help for his emotional problems. He asks you for your advice. When you assess Yuri's need for professional help, what symptoms do you look for?

____

____

____

____

____

6. Your friend, Maria, tells you that she has scheduled her first trip to a therapist. She seems to have misconceptions about what therapy is and how it works. What can you tell Maria to expect in the therapy sessions and what she can do to get the most out of therapy?

____

____

____

____

____

Critical Thinking Activity

Psychosocial health consists of mental, emotional, social, and spiritual health. In the space below, reflect on your own psychosocial health by defining each component of health in your own words.

Questions for the Critical Thinker

After you have completed the activity, reflect on the following questions. Your thoughtful responses will enhance your learning of this activity as well as your understanding of psychosocial health.

1. What component of psychosocial health is most developed in you? How have you enhanced this aspect of development?

2. What component of psychosocial health is least developed? What steps can you take to enhance this aspect of development?

3. What support systems do you have to help enhance your psychosocial health?

Language Enrichment Glossary

In addition to the words in the Key Terms list at the end of the chapter, students listed the following words as difficult to understand. Use the chapter Key Terms list, this list, your dictionary, and teachers and friends to learn the meaning of words you do not understand.

abscessed: enclosed, infected area
accreditation: licensing
acknowledge: admit to
adhere: stick to
adjuncts: additions
afflicted: affected by, bothered by
agitated: upset, disturbed
agonizing: highly painful
alterations: changes from original
apathy: indifference, passivity, low energy
apparent: appear to be, look as if
assess: examine and understand
bewilderment: confusion
black holes: slang for deep emotional depression
blank slate: small chalkboard without writing
boldest: most unusual
bombarded: being hit frequently by something
borderline: on the edge of something
brags: speak with pride about oneself
carbohydrate craving: strong desire for carbohydrates
chaos: disorder, unpredictability
cherish: value something greatly
clarify: make clear

conclusive: certain, convincing
contemplator: thinker
correlates: accompanies
credentials: certificates, qualifications
criterion: requirement, guideline
curb: limit
cynical: distrusting, expecting the worst
deteriorate: break down
devastated: destroyed
diagnosed: found the cause of
dietary deprivation: inadequate food or vitamins
diminish: make smaller
discord: disagreement
distorted: unrealistic, not accurate
emerge from: come out of
empathy: imagining how the other feels
encompasses: includes, surrounds
entails: requires
epidemic proportions: large numbers
execute: do something
exerted: effort towards, attempted
exhausted: extremely tired, worn out
fallacies: false, incorrect beliefs
fidelity: faithfulness
flaw: error
fluctuations: moving up and down
fosters: develops
gauge: measure
gender bias: prejudice against one gender
get your act together: behave sensibly, responsibly
grumpy: irritable, bad tempered
habitually: done regularly without thinking
hallmark: measure or symptom of
hallucinations: seeing things which are not real.
heart palpitations: not regular heart beats
hereditary: inherited
immediate gratification: prompt satisfaction of desires
immediate concern: more important worry
in conjunction: together
incremental: small steps toward something
inherently: basically, automatically
innate: inborn, inherited
integral: a central part of, indispensable
integration: being involved with, connected to
interfering: interrupting, getting in the way of
interpretations: explanations
intertwined: involved, wrapped around each other
intervention: attempt to stop something
intricately: delicately, in a complicated way
introverted: loner; focused on oneself
irrationally: not logically, without reason

lethargy: lack of energy, passivity
life span: expected years to live
lingering: continuing
linkages: connections
lounging: relaxing
lull: calm, soothe
manifestations: appearances
menopause: when menstrual cycles end in mid-life
metropolitan: associated with a city
mimic: imitate
mind reader: someone who can see into another's mind
mood elevation: increased good feelings
nurturance: care and nourishment
onset: beginning
optimal: best, highest
outlook: expectation, point of view
outward: external
overwrought: extremely distressed
past lives therapy: imagining lives one lived previously
persistent: stubborn, doesn't stop
pervasive: widespread
phenomenon: event, occurrence
ponder: think, wonder about something
precepts: basic principles, beliefs
precursor: occurs before
premenstrual: before a menstrual period
presumption: assumption, expectation
prevalence: frequent existence
prospect: an expectation of something
provisional: temporary until it can be confirmed
provoke: cause something
rampant: frequent and widespread
raring to go: eager, excited to get started
reason: think something through
recurring: happening over and over
reflection: evidence of something
regressing: going backward
reimbursement: repayment
reinvigorate: restore energy
restrain: limit, hold back
sap: drain, wear out
scheme: plan
sedated: given drugs to calm
set hierarchical order: fixed pattern of importance
setback: a reverse in one's progress
shelter: housing, protection from the outdoors
sizing up: estimating
slumped: bent over, without energy
snap out of: leave suddenly
sort through: examine one by one
static: not changing

stifle:	limit, smother
stigma:	mark of shame
subtly:	not obviously, indirectly
succumbing:	giving in to, yielding to
suicide-prone:	likely to commit suicide
summon up:	gather together
superficial:	on the surface, not deep
support group:	people who help each other with a shared problem
suppress:	avoid thinking about something
surmised:	believed, assumed
take in stride:	handle or accept without problems
take the short trip off a bridge:	commit suicide
trampled upon:	treated without respect
traumas:	shocks, injuries
utterly:	completely
vicious circle:	a negative thing causing another
vital:	important
volatile mood swing:	rapid change from one emotion to another
ward off:	avoid, stop
zest:	enthusiasm, energy

CHAPTER 3
MANAGING STRESS: COPING WITH LIFE'S CHALLENGES

Chapter Overview

Stress is defined as our mental and physical responses to change and challenges in our lives. Positive stress, or eustress, presents the opportunity for personal growth and satisfaction, whereas negative stress, or distress, results in debilitative stress and strain. Although stress is inevitable, we can learn to recognize what causes distress and to anticipate our reactions. We can develop stress management techniques.

Developing stress management skills depends on our understanding of the major components of stress with a similar physiological reaction known as the *fight-or-flight* response. Hans Selye called this physiological response to stress the general adaptation syndrome, which has three distinct phases. The three phases of the general adaptation syndrome describe the physiological response to stress. In the alarm phase, homeostasis is disturbed and the brain prepares the body either to fight or to run away. In the resistance phase, the body has reacted to the stressor and begins to allow the system to return to normal. In the exhaustion phase, the physical and psychological energy used to fight the stressors has been depleted. We can diminish the effects of stress by use of our *adaptation energy stores*, the physical and mental foundations of our ability to cope with stress. Stress management is dependent on an ability to replenish superficial stores and conserve deep stores.

Psychoneuroimmunology analyzes the relationship between the mind's response to stress and the ability of the immune system to function effectively. Several studies support the relationship between increased stress levels and greater risk of disease.

There are three major sources of stress. These sources include psychosocial factors, such as changes, hassles, pressure, inconsistent goals and objectives, conflict, overload, and burnout; environmental stressors, such as natural disasters and background distressors; and self-imposed stress. Self-esteem, personality type and hardiness, self-efficacy, and control influence our ability to cope successfully with stressful situations.

College students experience numerous distressors, not just those related to academic achievement. College students may be especially vulnerable because they are in a period of developmental transition, facing several key developmental tasks. Some symptoms of stress overload include difficulty concentrating on and finishing tasks, disinterest in social activities, difficulty in maintaining an intimate relationship, and disinterest in sexual relationships. It is important to act promptly to reduce their impact. Most colleges offer stress management workshops through their health centers or student counseling departments.

Stress management consists primarily of finding balance in our lives. Dealing with stress involves assessing your stressors, changing your responses, and learning to cope. Downshifting, a conscious attempt to simplify one's life in an effort to reduce the stresses of modern living, has become a trend in the 1990s. Stress management skills involve managing emotional responses, learning mental coping strategies, using physical activity to alleviate stress, managing your time, and making the most of support groups. The popularity of stress management has brought about alternative stress management techniques, such as hypnosis, massage, meditation, and biofeedback.

Learning Objectives

1. Define stress and examine how stress may have direct and indirect effects on your immune system and on your overall health status.

2. Explain the three phases of the general adaptation syndrome and describe what happens physiologically when you experience a real or perceived threat.

3. Examine the health risks that may occur with chronic stress.

4. Discuss psychosocial, environmental, and self-imposed sources of stress. Examine ways in which you might reduce risks from these stressors or inoculate yourself from stressful solutions.

5. Examine how evolving societal expectations may cause new kinds of stress.

6. Examine the special stressors that affect college students and strategies for reducing risk.

7. Explore techniques for coping with unavoidable stress, reducing exposure to stress, and making optimum use of positive stressors to promote growth and enrich life experiences.

Key Terms

Fill in a brief definition to help you remember these terms.

stress ____________________

stressor ____________________

adjustment ____________________

strain ____________________

eustress ____________________

distress ____________________

psychoneuroimmunology (PNI) ____________________

homeostasis ____________________

adaptive response ____________________

general adaptation syndrome (GAS) ____________________

immunocompetence ____________________

conflict ____________________

overload ____________________

burnout ____________________

psychological hardiness ____________________

background distressors ____________________

cognitive stress system ____________________

downshifting ____________________

hypnosis ____________________

meditation ____________________

biofeedback ____________________

Short Answers

1. Distinguish between eustress and distress, and provide an example of each.

2. What are the phases of the general adaptation syndrome?

3. What is the science of psychoneuroimmunology?

4. What is burnout, and what occupations make a person susceptible to experiencing it?

5. What is environmental stress, and what are some examples of this type of stress in the last year throughout the world?

6. Characterize a psychologically hardy individual.

7. List five symptoms of stress overload.

8. How does stress inoculation help people cope with stress?

9. What is downshifting, and why are increasing numbers of people opting for it?

10. Identify and describe one consumer product or service designed to fight stress.

Critical Thinking Exercises

1. In what ways can you replenish your superficial adaptation energy stores, thereby conserving your deep stores?

2. If you experience test-taking anxiety, what are some steps to take before and during the exam to ease your anxiety?

3. Changing the way you think is a key element of stress management. Identify ways to reframe and provide personal examples of each reframe when applicable.

4. Reginald is preparing for his bar exam to practice law, and as a consequence, he is experiencing a great deal of distress. As a single father, he is struggling to balance the demands of studying and family obligations. How can he manage his time most effectively?

5. Who forms your support group? If you do not have a close support group, to whom can you go when you feel overwhelmed?

Critical Thinking Activity: Stress and the College Student

College students face a number of stressful situations, such as homesickness, financial worries, academic achievement, and relationship problems. What may be a form of eustress to one college student may be a source of distress to another. The purpose of this activity is to explore with other college students what is considered stressful and to share ideas for managing particular stressors.

Complete the survey on college-related stressors. Then, select five volunteers to take the survey. All volunteers need to be college students. Provide a copy of the survey to each volunteer and ask them to complete the survey individually. Then have a group discussion on ways to manage stress in college.

SURVEY ON COLLEGE-RELATED STRESSORS

Rank these common sources of college-related stressors from 1 to 15, with 1 being the most stressful for you and 15 being the least stressful.

__________ completing homework assignments

__________ taking an exam

__________ financial difficulties

__________ roommate conflict

__________ making friends

__________ homesickness

__________ going on a date

__________ answering a question in class

__________ balancing school/job

__________ keeping up your grades

__________ deciding on your major

__________ peer pressure

__________ managing time

__________ parental conflict

__________ friend conflict

Questions for the Critical Thinker

After you have completed the survey, reflect on the following questions. Your thoughtful responses will enhance your learning from this activity as well as your understanding of managing stress.

1. How did your rankings of stress-related events compare with the rankings of others?

2. Successfully meeting the stressful tasks related to college is a form of growth-producing eustress. Identify such tasks that have been a form of eustress for you.

3. Both eustress and distress have many sources, including psychosocial factors, environmental stressors, and self-imposed stress. Identify personal sources of stress related to attending college.

4. What causes the most stress in your life? What in your own behavior increases your stress? What do you do to relieve the stress?

5. What components of stress management can help you achieve balance in college?

Language Enrichment Glossary

In addition to the words in the Key Terms list at the end of the chapter, students listed the following words as difficult to understand. Use the chapter Key Terms list, this list, your dictionary, and teachers and friends to learn the meaning of words you do not understand.

adversaries: competitors, enemies
alleviate: smooth, ease
anonymity: not being known
appraisal: judgment
by-products: things which result from
categorize: place things in similar groups
circumstances: characteristics of a situation
clergy: ministers and priests
clutching: holding tightly
cramping: painful muscle tightening
debilitative: damaging, destructive
deviate: change from
dilates: expands
disgruntled: annoyed, dissatisfied
dismiss: ignore, remove
disproportionately: stronger than expected
dissipate: lessen or eliminate
don't sweat the small stuff: don't be bothered by small things
elicited: brought up by
engendered: caused by
equilibrium: balance
exhaustion: extreme tiredness
fretting: worrying
gimmicks: tricks
gouge: to dig a hole into
hardiness: strength
hostile: angry towards others
impact: influence of
impetus: motivation
imposed: forced upon
inevitable: cannot be avoided
inhibiting: restricting, slowing
intangible: doesn't exist physically
intolerant: not willing to put up with something
legitimacy: accuracy, correctness
locus: place, center
manifest: appear
manifestation: occurrence
mediating factors: things which lessen a problem
migraines: very strong headaches
modification: change in something
onslaught: attack
potential: possible
psyches: minds, egos
reputable: honorable, responsible

restorative:	creating health and well-being
rev up:	slang for increase speed of operation
screeches:	screams in a high tone of voice
self-imposed:	created by the self
speculate:	guess
stamina:	strength, ability to continue
status:	standing
stewing:	thinking often about something
strained:	difficult to maintain
stress-tabs:	vitamins to reduce the effects of stress
stuttering:	talk slowed by inability to pronounce words smoothly
sustain:	experience, suffer
switch:	replace with something else
tangible:	actual, physically exist
terminal:	deadly
theorize:	suggest, assume
untangle:	clarify
web:	net
weed out trivia:	eliminate unimportant things

CHAPTER 4
INTENTIONAL AND UNINTENTIONAL INJURIES: STAYING SAFE IN A VIOLENT WORLD

Chapter Overview

The term violence is used to indicate a set of behaviors that produces injuries, regardless of whether they are intentional or unintentional. In 1985, the U.S. Public Health Service labeled violence as a leading public health problem that was contributing to significant death and disability rates among Americans. Several factors lead to violence and abuse, including poverty, unemployment, parental influence, cultural beliefs, the media, discrimination/oppression, religious differences, breakdowns in the criminal justice system, and stress. Anger and substance abuse also seem to be related to increased risk for violence. There are many forms of intentional violence. Homicide accounts for nearly 21,000 premature deaths every year in the United States. As the U.S. population becomes more diverse, there has been a corresponding rise in intolerance. It is believed that much of intolerance is caused by a fear of change and a desire to blame others when forces such as the economy and crime seem to be out of control. The growing influence of street gangs has had a harmful impact on the health of our country.

Domestic violence refers to the use of force to control and maintain power over another person in the home environment. It includes both actual harm as well as the threat of harm. The cycle of violence theory explains how women get caught in a downward spiral of domestic violence including abuse, contrition, further abuse, denial, and contrition that sometimes ends in deadly force. Child abuse includes sexual, psychological, or physical harm of a child by a caregiver.

Sexual violence against women is of epidemic proportions in this country. A growing body of research shows that sexual assault is encouraged by the normal socialization processes that males experience daily. College students are particularly vulnerable to date rape. Certain social assumptions prevent the realization of the true nature of sexual assault by both the perpetrator and the wider public, including minimization, trivialization, blaming the victim, and "boys will be boys." Sexual harassment is defined as any form of unwanted sexual attention.

Individuals can learn self-defense tactics that should lower a person's risk for assault. Prevention of violence begins with keeping yourself out of dangerous situations. There are several precautions you can take to lower your risk against rape, to prevent assaults at home, on the street, and in your car.

Learning Objectives

1. Differentiate between intentional and unintentional injuries and discuss societal and personal factors that contribute to violence in American society.

2. Identify those factors that contribute to homicide, domestic violence, sexual victimization, and other intentional acts of violence.

3. Identify strategies for prevention and risk reduction of intentional injuries.

4. Identify major areas of crime that are common on college campuses today and explain ways in which the campus community, law enforcement officials, and individuals can prevent crime from occurring.

5. Discuss the impact of unintentional injuries on American society and explain actions that might contribute to personal risks from injuries of all types.

Key Terms
Fill in a brief definition to help you remember these terms.

violence ________________________________

homicide ________________________________

domestic violence ________________________________

child abuse ________________________________

sexual abuse of children ________________________________

sexual assault ________________________________

rape ________________________________

sexual harassment ________________________________

intentional injuries________________________________

unintentional injuries________________________________

primary aggression________________________________

reactive aggression________________________________

Short Answers

1. Identify antecedents of violence.

2. Define domestic violence.

3. Identify and describe the three phases of Lenore Walker's cycle of violence.

4. What is the single greatest cause of injury to women in the United States today?

5. Define sexual harassment.

6. Identify four social assumptions that prevent the realization of the true nature of sexual assault by both the perpetrator and the wider public.

7. Summarize the research that suggests sexual assault is encouraged by the normal socialization processes that males experience daily.

Critical Thinking Exercises

1. You have just been elected to city council. One issue on the forum is how to prevent violence. What community strategies will you want to adopt for preventing violence?

____

____

____

____

____

2. It is believed that much of intolerance stems from a fear of change and a desire to blame others when forces such as the economy and crime seem to be out of control. What can you do personally to prevent bias and hate crimes?

3. Suppose you are the director of a youth program based in a gang-controlled neighborhood. What would you do to prevent young people from joining a gang?

4. Amanda was sexually harassed by her boss. When Amanda asked her boss a question about a report she was dictating, her boss commented on the size of her breasts. What actions should she take to prevent repeated sexual harassment and to help herself?

5. If a woman has just been the victim of a rape, what should she do to help herself?

6. Kay is a single woman who has just moved into a new neighborhood. What precautions should Kay take to avoid being assaulted in her home?

7. Sheralee is a freshman college student who commutes 60 miles daily to attend college classes. What steps can she take to prevent assaults in her car?

Critical Thinking Activity: The Impact of Television Violence

In this chapter, you learned about the epidemic of violence in this country. Violence is defined as a set of behaviors that produce injuries, as well as the outcomes of these behaviors (the injuries themselves). Some have raised the issue of whether violence on television contributes to violence in society at large.

This activity is designed to help you determine for yourself the impact of television violence. Observe three 15-minute segments of the following types of television shows: a) a cartoon show for children; b) a news report; and c) a prime time show. As you watch each television segment, record the frequency, type, and duration of violent behaviors that you observe. After watching the segments, respond to the following critical thinking questions.

Questions for the Critical Thinker

After you have completed watching the television segments, reflect on the following questions. Your thoughtful responses will enhance your learning from this activity as well as encourage understanding of the impact of television violence.

1. Compare and contrast each television segment on the frequency, type, and duration of violence observed.

2. Which television segment contained the greatest amount of violent acts?

3. Did these shows portray the consequences of the violent acts (e.g., people's grief over losing a loved one who had been murdered)?

4. At what age group were these shows aimed?

5. Could these shows have been presented equally well without showing violence?

6. Why do you think people are drawn to viewing violence?

7. Do you think prolonged exposure to violent acts makes one desensitized to violence?

8. Should television violence be regulated by the government? If so, how?

Language Enrichment Glossary

In addition to the words in the Key Terms list at the end of the chapter, students listed the following words as difficult to understand. Use the chapter Key Terms list, this list, your dictionary, and teachers and friends to learn the meaning of words you do not understand.

apt:	likely
boost:	lift
brutalized:	treated very roughly
callow:	immature
carjackings:	stealing someone's car while he or she is in it
coax:	persuade
coitus interruptus:	sex without orgasm
conviction:	belief
crest and break:	rise and fall
desecration:	dishonor
deviance:	abnormal, unhealthy
discern:	see
douche:	wash the vagina
dynamics:	interaction
empathic:	able to imagine how the other feels
etiology:	causes
flip on:	turn on
forestall:	prevent
foster:	encourage
hindsight:	making judgments afterwards
impunity:	without punishment
intent:	focused
interact:	be involved
intolerance:	prejudice
jocular:	funny
lurking:	hiding
millennia:	thousands of years
minimization:	to make smaller
objectify:	seen as an object
odds:	chances
perpetrated:	caused
plagiarism:	taking credit for another's work
ploys:	tricks
precipitated:	caused
punitive:	harsh punishment
rash:	increased occurrence
relative:	in comparison
retaliation:	revenge
rife:	full
self-righteousness:	believing you are right
stifle:	push down
streaking:	running naked past a group
systematic:	repeated process
toxic:	poisonous
trivialization:	to make unimportant
vigilant:	watchful

CHAPTER 5
COMMUNICATING EFFECTIVELY: A KEY TO INTERPERSONAL HEALTH

Chapter Overview

Good communication skills contribute significantly to your mental, emotional, spiritual, social, and physical dimensions of health. Communication is the transmission of information and meaning from one individual to another. Communication is only successful when both parties understand not only the information communicated, but also the meaning of that information. There are many barriers to communication. For instance, common barriers between patients and medical practitioners include language specialization, issues of power and control, sociocultural differences, and patient anxiety. However, both patient and practitioner can help to remove barriers. Self-disclosure is the sharing of personal information with others.

Because listening is such a vital part of our interpersonal communication, it is important that we develop good listening skills. Listening involves paying attention to nonverbal communication. If there is a contradiction between what a person says and what he or she does, we tend to believe the nonverbal messages.

One common method for improving communication with others is learning to use "I" messages (e.g., "I like being with you," "I am sorry.") The basic premise of using "I" messages is that each individual takes responsibility for communicating his or her own feelings. Communicating assertively means using direct, honest communication that maintains and defends your rights in a positive manner, while respecting the rights of others. It is important to consider your actions in establishing a proper climate for an open, honest conversation. This is more likely to happen if you avoid judgmental statements, keep an open mind, avoid projecting superiority, don't ask for feedback unless you want an honest answer, and avoid people who tend to give negative feedback. Most conflicts revolve around content and relationship. Conflict resolution can be a growth process as we learn to recognize problems and solutions based upon past experience.

Differences in communication styles make communication between the genders confusing and difficult. Psychologist Deborah Tannen coined the term *genderlect* to characterize very real differences in word choices, interruption patterns, questioning patterns, language interpretations and misinterpretations, and vocal influences based on gender. Communication in intimate relationships between two adults is often a source of difficulty. Techniques which can help improve communication between couples include leveling (sending your partner a clear, simple and honest message), editing (censoring remarks that are meant to be hurtful), documenting (providing specific examples), and validating (letting your partner know that although you may disagree with him/her, you still respect his/her thoughts and feelings.)

Learning Objectives

1. Discuss the impact that good communication skills can have on your health, including improved self-esteem, reduced stress, and increased health knowledge.

2. Discuss the process of communication, including barriers that inhibit successful communication, such as differences in background, substance abuse, language and culture, and issues of power and control and anxiety.

3. Explain the importance of trusting others enough to be able to let others be themselves.

4. Discuss the importance of effective listening and speaking skills in verbal and nonverbal communication and the ways in which you can improve your own skills in these areas.

5. Explain ways in which you can improve your communication skills through the use of "I" messages, assertive communication, establishing proper climates, and resolving conflicts.

6. Compare and contrast the communication styles of men and women, and discuss actions that you might take to help reduce potential problems.

Key Terms

Fill in a brief definition to help you remember these terms.

communication ____________________

self-disclosure ____________________

nonverbal communication ____________________

"I" messages ____________________

assertive communicators ____________________

nonassertive communicators ____________________

aggressive communicators ____________________

conflict ____________________

conflict resolution ____________________

genderlect ____________________

leveling ____________________

editing ____________________

documenting ____________________

validating ____________________

alexithymia____________________

risk communication____________________

Short Answers

1. Identify the five parts of the communication process.

2. What risk is involved in not disclosing yourself to others?

3. List barriers to listening.

4. How can you keep your listening in the present?

5. Distinguish between an "I" message and a "you" message. Illustrate the difference between each message.

6. What are the typical verbal and nonverbal behaviors of nonassertive communicators?

7. What steps should a person take in order to establish a proper climate for communication?

8. Most conflicts revolve around what two message components?

Critical Thinking Exercises

1. Andre has been diagnosed with high blood pressure and high cholesterol. He complains that his doctor uses words that he doesn't understand and that he talks "over his head." Andre doesn't always follow his doctor's advice about diet and exercise because he says that the doctor gives him so much information that he is overwhelmed and cannot remember all of his instructions. What can Andre do to remove barriers to communication?

____

____

____

____

____

2. Elliot has been your best friend for 10 years. Now he comes to you for advice. He confides that his girlfriend is frustrated with him because he won't "open up" and share his true feelings. What would help Elliot overcome his fears of self-disclosure?

____

____

____

____

____

3. Malcolm has gotten into the habit of not always listening to what his roommate is saying. He has also found himself daydreaming in classes and being called on by the instructor, only to sheepishly admit that he wasn't paying attention. After being embarrassed repeatedly, Malcolm decides to work on improving his listening skills. What methods can help him become a better listener?

____

____

____

____

____

4. Your spouse has repeatedly called your boss complaining that you are not paid enough, that you have more work than anyone else in your department, and has even suggested that your boss is incompetent. Now your boss has told you that if these calls continue, you will be fired. How would you discuss this with your spouse using "I" instead of "you" messages?

____

____

____

____

____

5. Linda is worried about her husband, Al. Al's father died recently, and he has not cried or talked about his feelings. You are consulted to explain Al's behavior to Linda. What would you tell her, based on your knowledge about gender differences in communication styles?

____

____

____

____

____

6. Married just over two years, Sara and Jim are having a rough time. They have just about given up talking about sex, money, careers, in-laws, and children. Trying to talk about any of these subjects leads to fighting and bad feelings. What techniques can Sara and Jim use to improve their communication?

____

____

____

____

____

Critical Thinking Activity: The Impact of Role Models

Lack of adequate role models may also be a barrier to good communication. Most of us learn the basics of communicating with others by watching and listening to those around us. Think back to your parents, your aunts and uncles, your teachers, and your other adult role models. How did these role models affect the way you communicate? What other role models did you have? Did sports or entertainment figures affect how you communicate? Do you think children today have fewer role models? If so, why?

Language Enrichment Glossary

In addition to the words in the Key Terms list at the end of the chapter, students listed the following words as difficult to understand. Use the Key Terms list, this list, your dictionary, and teachers and friends to learn the meaning of words you do not understand.

absolute:	definite, unquestioned
accusatory:	blaming the other
alienation:	become unfriendly, isolated from another
aspects:	features
bruises:	injuries in which the skin is discolored
concerted:	focused
crummy:	not good quality
curable:	able to be cured
decodes:	to take meaning from words heard
detached:	not connected
differentiate:	notice the difference between
dilemmas:	problems, puzzles
diminish:	lessen
discern:	see, determine
double-edged sword:	has a good and a bad side
dredge up:	recall, bring to others' attention
dynamic:	continuously changing
embodies:	carries

encodes:	to put thoughts into words
erect:	straight, upright
escalating:	increasing
estranged:	isolated
evasive:	avoiding
ever-looming:	a threat always present
feedback:	answer, response
flaws:	faults, imperfections
gross:	broad, vague
hesitant:	reluctant, not willing
inflammatory:	tendency to make angry
innocuous:	harmless, not offensive
irrelevant:	not related
jargon:	technical terms
logical:	reasonable
loyalty:	faithfulness
mammogram:	x-ray to find breast cancer
mow:	to cut evenly
negotiate:	make a bargain
nonverbal:	any communication without words
optimistic:	hopeful, positive view
paraphrasing:	restating another's points in your own words
pessimistic:	hopeless, negative view
place at risk:	to put in a difficult situation
projecting:	giving an impression
rapport:	liking, good feeling toward others
resolve:	solve
ridiculous:	foolish
sappy:	slang for silly, foolish
selective:	carefully chosen
self-esteem:	how much an individual likes him or herself
soaring:	rapidly rising
stew over:	continue thinking about
subtle:	not obvious
suspect:	imagine
taboos:	social restrictions against something
tactic:	strategy, technique, approach
variables:	factors

CHAPTER 6
HEALTHY RELATIONSHIPS: FRIENDS, FAMILY, AND SIGNIFICANT OTHERS

Chapter Overview

Intimate relationships involve behavioral interdependence, need fulfillment, and emotional attachment. Each of these three characteristics may be related to interactions with family, close friends, and romantic partners.

Despite dramatic changes in the American family since the 1950s, all families still have in common the special bonding that a group of people with shared interests have for each other. Friendships are characterized by enjoyment, acceptance, trust, respect, mutual assistance, confiding, understanding, and spontaneity. Love relationships typically include all the characteristics of friendship, as well as fascination, exclusiveness, sexual desire, giving the utmost, and being an advocate. For Robert Sternberg, love is composed of three ingredients: intimacy, passion, and decision/commitment. According to Sternberg, the higher the levels of intimacy, passion, and commitment, the more likely a person is to be involved in a healthy, positive love relationship. Falling in love may be due to imprinting, attraction, attachment, and production of a cuddle chemical.

Gender differences in relating styles stem from our social conditioning. One theory about why males and females relate as they do is that men are less able to express emotions and achieve intimacy than are women, owing to the process of identity development in infancy, considered more difficult for males than for females. The process of partner selection also shows distinctly different patterns. Factors that play a significant role in partner selection include proximity, similarities, reciprocity, and physical attraction. Men tend to select their partners primarily on the basis of youth and physical attractiveness, whereas women tend to place higher emphasis on partners who are somewhat older, have good financial prospects, and are dependable and industrious.

Obstacles to intimacy include lack of personal identity, emotional immaturity, and a poorly developed sense of responsibility. Barriers to intimacy stem from the different emotional development of men and women, an upbringing in a dysfunctional family, or other causes.

Commitment in a relationship means that there is an intent to act over time in a way that perpetuates the well-being of the other person, yourself, and the relationship. What separates committed from uncommitted relationships is the willingness of committed partners to dedicate themselves to acquiring and using the skills that will ensure a lasting relationship. The major types of committed relationships are marriage, cohabitation, and gay and lesbian partnerships.

Success in committed relationships requires understanding the roles of partnering scripts. Accountability and self-nurturance are especially important in knowing yourself and maintaining a good relationship. People in healthy committed relationships trust one another, meaning there is predictability, dependability, and faith. Couples seeking a long-term relationship have to confront a number of issues, such as changing gender roles and power sharing, that can affect their chances of success.

More people are remaining single, either by choice or by chance. Many single people live rich, rewarding lives and maintain a large network of close friends and families.

Having children changes a couple's relationship. Resources of time, energy, and money are split many ways, and the partners no longer have each other's undivided attention. Consistency, communication, affection, and mutual respect are important to the well-being of the family unit.

usually difficult, and it often takes at least a year or longer to recover from the loss of a major relationship. With time, support from others, and community or professional help, most people do recover and establish new relationships.

Learning Objectives

1. Explain the characteristics of intimate relationships, the purposes they serve, and the types of intimacy that each of us may be able to have.

2. Explain how relationships develop and describe the factors that influence their formation and maintenance.

3. Discuss the differences between men and women when it comes to relationships, partner selection, and communication styles.

4. Discuss the barriers to intimate relationships and explain how these barriers can be overcome.

5. Discuss the importance of commitment, honesty, and mutual respect in each of the various types of relationships described.

6. Examine those factors that seem to be important in determining the success of an intimate relationship.

7. Discuss what remaining single means for many Americans.

8. Examine child-rearing practices in the United States and the importance of a healthy family environment.

9. Discuss the warning signs of relationship decline, where you can go to get help with a relationship crisis, and factors that ultimately lead to relationship problems.

10. Discuss what actions you can take to improve your own interpersonal interactions.

Key Terms

Fill in a brief definition to help you remember these terms.

intimate relationships ____________________

emotional availability ____________________

dysfunctional family ____________________

jealousy ____________________

monogamy ____________________

serial monogamy ____________________

open relationship ____________________

cohabitation ____________________

common-law marriage ______________________________

accountability ______________________________

self-nurturance ______________________________

trust ______________________________

autonomy ______________________________

power ______________________________

psychoeducation______________________________

Short Answers

1. What are three characteristics of an intimate relationship?

2. Regardless of the form or structure of each family, what unique characteristic do all families have in common?

3. The United Nations defines seven basic types of families. List them.

4. Identify four categories of significant sexual or committed relationships.

5. What are the characteristics of love relationships?

6. What three conditions must be met in order for passionate love to occur?

7. Describe the process of falling in love as explained by anthropologist Helen Fisher.

8. What factors play a significant role in selecting a partner? What similarities and differences exist between genders in the process of partner selection?

9. What is a common-law marriage?

10. Two concepts that are important to knowing yourself and maintaining a good relationship are accountability and self-nurturance. Define these concepts.

Critical Thinking Exercises

1. Bill and Debbie have been dating each other exclusively for two years. According to Lillian Rubin, what is the single greatest threat to intimacy in their relationship?

___

___

___

___

___

2. Every time Ben and Susan go to a party, Ben gets extremely jealous when Susan talks to other men. What are some possible causes of Ben's jealousy?

3. What is a partnering script? While growing up, what script were you raised with for what is expected of you as an adult? How does it influence your partner selection?

4. When Felipe explained to his parents that he trusts his fiancée, what did he mean?

5. Following her divorce from Andy, Sandy is experiencing great loneliness and an intense desire for new relationships. What steps can she take to cope effectively?

Critical Thinking Activity: Friendship Values

Psychologists Jeffrey Turner and Laurna Rubinson provide an overview of what characterizes friendships. Rank the following characteristics in terms of what you value most in a friendship. Then give the same handout to a good friend. After he or she has ranked the characteristics, compare your responses with each other.

CHARACTERISTICS OF FRIENDSHIP

Directions: Rank the following characteristics of a friendship in terms of what you value in a friendship. Rank from 1 to 8 (1 = most valued characteristic and 8 = least valued characteristic).

__________ enjoyment

__________ acceptance

__________ trust

__________ respect

__________ mutual assistance

__________ confiding

__________ understanding

__________ spontaneity

Questions for the Critical Thinker

After you and your friend have completed your ranking, reflect on the following questions. Your thoughtful responses will enhance your learning of this activity as well as your understanding of healthy relationships.

1. How did your responses compare with your friend's responses? What do you value the most in a friendship? What do you value the least?

2. How do these characteristics compare with those of an intimate relationship?

3. Are there any other characteristics not listed by Turner and Rubinson that you value in a friendship?

Language Enrichment Glossary

In addition to the words in the Key Terms list at the end of the chapter, students listed the following words as lifficult to understand. Use the chapter Key Terms list, this list, your dictionary, and teachers and friends to learn the neaning of words you do not understand.

gony: pain
limony: support payments after divorce
lleviate: reduce
nnoyance: irritation
pparently: likely, seems to
rena: area, topic
spects: different sides to something
ssume: expect, take for granted
ssumption: expectation
ttributes: characteristics
versive: strongly negative
elebrated: held in high esteem
hild-rearing practices: ways of raising children
ognitive: related to thought
ontradictory: conflicting, inconsistent
ornerstones: foundations
orporate ladder: levels of job status
iteria: measurement
uddle: hug, snuggle
erail: cause problems for a plan of action
signated: specified
trimental: harmful
mensions: areas

discernible:	separate, distinct
disparity:	contrast, difference
divulge:	to reveal, tell
dominant:	strongest influence
ecstasy:	joy
elaboration:	giving more details
elation:	joy, delight
eliciting:	bringing up
equated:	associated with
evoke:	bring up, remind
evolve:	develop
exclusiveness:	limited to one person
exerted:	to put forward
fascination:	to have strong interest in
flaws:	imperfections
formation:	development
frantic:	agitated, extremely upset
frowns:	looks down upon, discourages
grooming:	personal cleanliness
hostility:	hate, anger
incentives:	encouragements
infatuation:	obsession, preoccupation
infidelity:	unfaithfulness
inhibits:	slows down, holds back
insemination:	to become pregnant
integration:	union with others
intertwined:	involved with each other
introspection:	self-analysis
junkies:	people addicted to something
justified:	defended, excused
love-smitten:	captivated by love
matrimony:	marriage
mutual:	shared both ways
norm:	average
offset:	help to balance
opt:	choose
perpetuates:	continues
postpone:	do it later
precludes:	prevents
prelude:	beginning
pristine:	perfect
provocative:	interesting, intriguing
provoke:	cause
proximity:	nearness
punctuated:	emphasized, highlighted
quadrupled:	increased 400%
reciprocal:	mutual, shared
reciprocity:	return similar behavior
recur:	happen over and over
refute:	contradict
resilient:	strong, flexible

rivalry:	competition
sanctioned:	approved
scripting:	habitual behavior
shed light:	reveal
siblings:	brothers and sisters
soaring:	rising rapidly
solidify:	make stronger
speculate:	guess, imagine
spontaneity:	action without planning
stem:	come from
stigma:	shame
surrogate:	substitute
sustain:	maintain, continue over time
theme:	focus, subject
traits:	characteristics
ultimately:	finally
unsolicited:	unasked
utmost:	maximum
validation:	support for, confirmed
verbalize:	say
vital:	necessary
void:	absence, empty space
wading:	moving slowly through something

CHAPTER 7
SEXUALITY: DEFINING YOUR SEXUAL BEHAVIOR

Chapter Overview

Your sexual identity is determined by a complex interaction of genetic, physiological, and environmental factors. Defining your sexual identity is a lifelong process of growing and learning. Your sexual identity is made up of the unique combination of your sex, gender identity, chosen gender roles, sexual preference, and personal experiences.

An understanding of the female and male reproductive systems will help you derive pleasure and satisfaction from your sexual relationships, be sensitive to your partner's wants and needs, and be more responsible about your choices regarding your own sexual health. The female reproductive system includes the mons pubis, the labia minora and majora, the clitoris, the urethral and vaginal openings, the vestibule of the vagina, vagina, uterus, fallopian tubes, and ovaries. The male reproductive system includes the penis, scrotum, testes, epididymides, vasa deferentia, urethra, the seminal vesicles, the prostate gland, and the Cowper's glands.

For both males and females, the human sexual response is a physiological process that involves four stages: excitement/arousal, plateau, orgasm, and resolution. The response stages occur during masturbation, heterosexual activity, and homosexual activity. Sexual orientation refers to a person's enduring emotional, romantic, sexual or affectionate attraction to other persons. Sexual orientation is categorized by heterosexuality, homosexuality, and bisexuality. The range of human sexual expression is broad, such as celibacy, autoerotic behaviors, kissing and erotic touching, oral-genital stimulation, vaginal intercourse, and anal intercourse. Variant sexual behaviors are sexual behaviors that are not engaged in by most people, such as group sex and transvestitism.

Various problems associated with achieving sexual satisfaction are called sexual dysfunctions. Sexual dysfunctions include sexual desire disorders, sexual arousal disorders, orgasm disorders, and sexual pain disorders. Various drug use can also lead to sexual dysfunction. Many theories and treatment models exist for those seeking help for sexual dysfunctions. Of growing concern in recent years is the increasing use of " date-rape drugs."

Learning Objectives

1. Identify the components of male and female reproductive anatomy and physiology and their functions.

2. Discuss the options available for the expression of one's sexuality.

3. Classify sexual dysfunctions and describe each disorder.

4. Define sexual identity and discuss the roles of the major components of sexual identity, including biological sex, gender identity, gender roles and sexual orientation.

Key Terms

Fill in a brief definition to help you remember these terms.

sexual identity ____

gonads ____

puberty ____

pituitary gland ____ secondary sex characteristics ____________________

vasocongestion ____________________

cervix ____________________

ovaries ____________________

fallopian tubes ____________________

puberty ____________________

pituitary gland ____________________

hypothalamus ____________________

gonadotropin-releasing hormone (GnRH) ____________________

follicle-stimulating hormone (FSH) ____________________

luteinizing hormone (LH) ____________________

estrogens ____________________

progesterone ____________________

menarche ____________________

ovarian follicles (egg sacs) ____________________

ovulation ____________________

human chorionic gonadotropin (HCG) ____________________

menopause ____________________

external male genitals ____________________

internal male genitals ____________________

accessory glands ____________________

penis ____________________

gender ____________________

gender roles ____________________

gender identity ____________________

gender role stereotypes ____________________

androgyny ____

socialization ____

external female genitals ____

vulva ____

mons pubis ____

labia minora ____

labia majora ____

clitoris ____

urethral opening ____

vagina ____

hymen ____

perineum ____

internal female genitals ____

uterus (womb) ____

endometrium ____

ejaculation ____

scrotum ____

testes ____

testosterone ____

spermatogenesis ____

epididymis ____

vas deferens ____

seminal vesicles ____

semen ____

prostate gland ____

foreskin ______________________________

sexual orientation ______________________________

heterosexual ______________________________

homosexual ______________________________

bisexual ______________________________

homophobia ______________________________

celibacy ______________________________

autoerotic behaviors ______________________________

sexual fantasies ______________________________

masturbation ______________________________

erogenous zones ______________________________

cunnilingus ______________________________

fellatio ______________________________

anal intercourse ______________________________

vaginal intercourse ______________________________

variant sexual behavior ______________________________

sexual dysfunction ______________________________

inhibited sexual desire (ISD) ______________________________

sexual aversion disorder ______________________________

erectile dysfunction ______________________________

impotence ______________________________

premature ejaculation ______________________________

female orgasmic disorder ______________________________

dyspareunia ______________________________

vaginismus ______________________________

Short Answers

1. How is an individual's sexual identity determined?

2. Identify secondary sex characteristics in males and in females.

3. Identify the external genitals and the internal genitals of the female reproductive system.

4. Identify and describe the three phases of the menstrual cycle.

5. Identify the external genitals and the internal genitals of the male reproductive system.

6. Identify four stages of the sexual response cycle.

7. Define sexual orientation. What are three forms of such orientation?

8. Identify and discuss various forms of sexual expression.

9. Identify and define three forms of variant sexual behaviors.

10. What is the most frequent problem that causes people to seek out a sex therapist?

Critical Thinking Exercises

1. Recall your own childhood. How were gender roles shaped or socialized by your parents, other family members, peers, schools, textbooks, advertisements, television, music, and movies?

____

____

____

____

____

2. The text identifies characteristics of sexually healthy adults. Which of these aspects of sexual health do you possess? Which of these aspects do you feel you need to work on?

____

____

____

____

____

3. Match the following sexual dysfunctions with the descriptions that follow.

a. inhibited sexual desire
b. vaginismus
c. dyspareunia
d. premature ejaculation
e. erectile dysfunction
f. female orgasmic disorder
g. sexual aversion disorder

_____ 1. When Lateefah was a child, she was sexually abused by her stepfather. As an adult, Lateefah experiences a great deal of anxiety about sexual contact.

_____ 2. Janet is seeking out a sex therapist because she doesn't have any interest in sexual activity.

_____ 3. Julia seeks out a sex therapist because she is unable to achieve orgasm.

_____ 4. Marco is experiencing difficulty in maintaining a penile erection for intercourse. His urologist asks him if he is still taking medication for high blood pressure.

_____ 5. Anthony goes to his urologist for a physical examination and complains of ejaculating soon after the insertion of the penis into the vagina.

_____ 6. Sarita has experienced pain during intercourse since she was diagnosed with endometriosis.

_____ 7. Bev's gynecologist explained to her that her fear of intercourse is most likely contributing to the involuntary contraction of vaginal muscles, making penile insertion painful.

4. What are "date-rape drugs" and how can you prevent exposure to such drugs?

____

____

____

____

____

Critical Thinking Activity: Assessing Your Sexuality

In order to evaluate your attitudes toward sexuality, complete the following sentences.

1. My definition of masculinity is ______________________________

____

2. My definition of femininity is ______________________________

____

3. I think my body is ______________________________

____

4. My sexual experiences have been ______________________________

____

5. My parents' attitudes toward sex ______________________________

____

6. A healthy sexual relationship is ______________________________

____

7. Homosexuality is ______________________________

____

8. When it comes to talking about sex with my partner, I ______________________________

____

9. Regarding male and female reproductive anatomy, my knowledge is ______________________________

____

10. My feelings about variant sexual behaviors are ______________________________

____

Language Enrichment Glossary

In addition to the words in the Key Terms list at the end of the chapter, students listed the following words as difficult to understand. Use the Key Terms list, this list, your dictionary, and teachers and friends to learn the meaning of words you do not understand.

abdomen:	stomach area
abnormalities:	things which are not normal
abound:	exist in large numbers
anatomical:	related to the body structure
anesthetic:	drug to lessen pain
chanting:	singing or speaking in one tone
coarse:	rough, not smooth
delineated:	defined, outlined
deviant:	different from normal
dwelling:	thinking often about something
erotic:	sexually stimulating
erroneously:	incorrectly
fraternal twins:	twins from separate eggs
gratification:	satisfaction
implantation:	act of inserting something
inanimate:	not alive
incest:	sexual relations with a close blood relative
introspection:	reviewing one's own thoughts and feelings
intrusive:	distracting, annoying
lesbians:	women sexually attracted to other women
lubricate:	to become slippery
nurturing:	caring for
pathological:	disorder in behavior, disease
penile:	related to the penis
prenatal:	before birth
rhythmic:	a recurring pattern
secrete:	release
sloughed off:	dropped off the top layer
socioeconomic:	social and economic standing
sort out:	separate, place in order
spur:	cause, act as a stimulus
succinctly:	briefly, directly
trigger mechanism:	something that causes something else
triggered:	caused
vastly:	enormously
via:	by or through

CHAPTER 8
BIRTH CONTROL, PREGNANCY, AND CHILDBIRTH: MANAGING YOUR FERTILITY

Chapter Overview

Conception refers to the fertilization of an ovum by a sperm. In order for conception to occur, there must be a viable egg, a viable sperm, and access to the egg by the sperm. Contraception refers to methods of preventing conception. The *perfect failure rate* and the *typical use failure rate* allows us to evaluate the efficacy of a particular contraceptive method. Reversible methods of contraception include abstinence and "outercourse," the condom, oral contraceptives, progestin-only pills, emergency contraceptives, foams, suppositories, jellies, and creams, the female condom, the diaphragm with spermicidal jelly or cream, the cervical cap, intrauterine devices, and withdrawal. New methods of birth control include Depo-Provera and Norplant. A method that is not yet approved by the FDA is the vaginal ring, which has an effectiveness rate similar to the pill. Researchers are working on new male contraceptives. Fertility awareness methods include the cervical mucous method, body temperature method, and the calendar method. Tubal ligation is a method of sterilization in females, and a procedure called a vasectomy is used for sterilization in males.

An abortion is the medical means of terminating a pregnancy. In 1973, the landmark Supreme Court decision in *Roe v. Wade* ruled that during the first trimester of pregnancy, a woman and her practitioner have the right to terminate the pregnancy through abortion without legal restrictions and allowed individual states to set conditions for second-trimester abortions. In July 1989, in *Webster v. Reproductive Health Services*, the Supreme Court gave states the right to impose certain new restrictions on abortions. The type of abortion procedure used is determined by the duration of the pregnancy.

The decision to become a parent involves a number of considerations, including your emotional health, maternal and paternal health, finances, and contingency planning.

Good prenatal care is essential for a successful pregnancy. Regular medical checkups, beginning as early in the pregnancy as possible, are essential. Other factors that contribute to a successful pregnancy include the availability of a skilled medical practitioner, the mother's avoidance of drugs and medication, her avoidance of X-rays, and good nutrition and exercise. Pregnancy typically lasts 40 weeks and is divided into three trimesters, of approximately three months each. A number of prenatal testing and screening procedures are able to detect health defects in a fetus, including amniocentesis, ultrasound, fetoscopy, and chorionic villus sampling.

There are three stages in the birth process. In the first stage, the amniotic sac breaks, causing a rush of fluid from the vagina. Contractions push the baby downward, causing the cervix to dilate further. When the cervix is sufficiently dilated, the second stage begins. During expulsion, uterine contractions push the baby through the birth canal. Expulsion concludes when the infant is finally pushed out of the mother's body. The third stage, afterbirth, occurs when the placenta is expelled from the womb, usually within thirty minutes after delivery. In addition to the traditional hospital birth, there are a number of alternatives available today, including the Lamaze method, the Harris method, childbirth without fear, and the Leboyer method. Problems and complications can occur during labor and delivery, even following a successful pregnancy. Such possibilities should be discussed with the medical practitioner prior to labor so that the mother understands what medical procedures may be necessary for her safety and for that of her child.

Approximately one in six American couples experience difficulty in conceiving. Reasons for infertility include the trend toward delaying childbirth and the rise in the incidence of pelvic inflammatory disease. Endometriosis is the leading cause of infertility in women in the United States, while low sperm count is the single largest fertility problem among men. There are a number of options available to couples with fertility problems, including fertility drugs, alternative insemination, in vitro fertilization, gamete intrafallopian transfer, intracytoplasmic sperm injection, nonsurgical embryo transfer, embryo transfer, embryo freezing, embryo adoption programs, surrogate motherhood, and adoption. Overall success rates for fertility treatments range from 30 to 70 percent, depending on the specific cause of the infertility.

Learning Objectives

1. List permanent and reversible contraceptive methods, discuss their effectiveness in preventing pregnancy and sexually transmitted diseases, and describe how these methods are used.

2. Summarize the legal decisions surrounding abortion and the various types of abortion procedures used today.

3. Discuss emotional health, maternal health, financial evaluation, and contingency planning in terms of your own life's goals as aspects that you should consider before becoming a parent.

4. Explain the importance of prenatal care and the process of pregnancy.

5. Describe the basic stages of childbirth as well as some of the complications that can arise during labor and delivery.

6. Review some of the primary causes of and possible solutions to infertility.

Key Terms

Fill in a brief definition to help you remember these terms.

Body temperature method Menstural cycle, monitor ovulation

Calendar method Monitor for ovulation

Sterilization Visectimay (vas deferens), tubaligation (ova

Oral contraceptives Pills

Fertility awareness methods (FAM) check ovulation

Cervical mucus method checking for ovulation

Vacuum aspiration ______

Dilation and evacuation (D&E) Sucked out

Dilation and curettage (D&C) stirred + then sucked/scrape

Hysterotomy removal of fetus

Induction abortion ~~0.4 - 0.8 Death~~ Chemicals used to abor

RU-486 abortion pill

Preconception care Pre-natal care

Toxic shock syndrome bacteria caused

Cervical cap fits over cervix

Intrauterine device (IUD) Coil, string method in Uterus

Withdrawal removing penis before ejaculation

Depo-Provera Birth control, last for 3 months

Norplant 6 capsules planted in arm

Emergency contraceptive pills (ECPs) taken within 3 days of sex

Spermicides kills sperm

Female condom made out of latex, 3 cervical rings

Diaphragm Dome shaped, birth control, by Dr.

Fertility produce sperm or eggs

Conception egg + sperm unite.

Contraception any form of birth control

Condom form of birth control made of latex

Tubal ligation cutting of flopian tube

Hysterectomy uterus taken out

Vasectomy Vas defrense taken out

Abortion Removal of fetus, Killing of fetus

Teratogenic taking something that causes birth defects

Fetal alcohol syndrome (FAS) Infant born to Mom that drank alcohol

Postpartum depression

Cesarean section (C-section)

Miscarriage fetus aborts by itself

Rh factor Rh+ Dominant over Rh−

Ectopic pregnancy

Stillbirth

Down's syndrome____

Afterbirth____

Transition____

Episiotomy____

Perineum____

Infertility____

Pelvic inflammatory disease (PID)____

Endometriosis____

Low sperm count____

Fertility drugs____

Alternative insemination____

In vitro fertilization____

Human chorionic gonadotropin (HCG)____

Trimester____

Embryo____

Fetus____

Placenta____

Amniocentesis____

Amniotic sac____

Gamete intrafallopian transfer (GIFT)____

Intracytoplasmic sperm injection (ICSI)____

Nonsurgical embryo transfer____

Embryo transfer____

Embryo freezing____

Embryo adoption programs____

Short Answers

1. What three conditions are necessary for conception?

(1)

(2)

(3)

2. Match the reversible method of contraception with its definition.

a. abstinence
b. outercourse
c. condom
d. spermicides
e. female condom
f. diaphragm
g. cervical cap
h. oral contraceptives
i. progestin-only pills
j. emergency contraceptive pill
k. intrauterine device
l. Depo-Provera

_____ 1. chemical substances that kill sperm

_____ 2. a small cup made of latex that is designed to fit snugly over the entire cervix

_____ 3. deliberately shunning intercourse

_____ 4. pills taken daily for 3 weeks of the menstrual cycle to prevent ovulation through regulation of hormones

_____ 5. a sheath of thin latex designed to fit over an erect penis and catch semen upon ejaculation

_____ 6. oral-genital sex and mutual masturbation

_____ 7. a soft, shallow cup made of thin latex rubber designed to fit snugly behind the pubic bone in front of the cervix and over the back of the cervix on the other side and used with spermicidal cream or jelly

_____ 8. an injectable method of birth control that lasts for three months

_____ 9. single-use, loose-fitting polyurethane sheath designed as one unit with two diaphragm-like rings

_____ 10. mini-pills that contain small doses of progesterone

_____ 11. pill can be used immediately after unprotected intercourse, and up to 72 hours beyond

_____ 12. a T-shaped plastic device that is implanted in the uterus to prevent conception

3. What are the procedures for female and male sterilization?

4. What are early signs of pregnancy?

5. Match the following prenatal procedure with its purpose.

a. fetoscopy
b. amniocentesis
c. ultrasound
d. chorionic villi sampling

_____ 1. This procedure reveals the presence of 40 genetic abnormalities, as well as the sex of the child.

_____ 2. This procedure determines the size and position of the fetus and can also detect defects in the central nervous system and digestive system of the fetus.

_____ 3. This procedure allows viewing the fetus directly.

_____ 4. This procedure involves snipping tissue from the developing fetal sac for couples who are at high risk for having a baby with Down's syndrome or a debilitating hereditary disease.

6. What are the three stages in the birth process?

7. What are reasons for performing a cesarean section? Once a woman has had a cesarean section, must all subsequent deliveries also be cesarean?

8. What percentage of American couples experience difficulty conceiving? What are causes of infertility for women? For men?

Critical Thinking Exercises

1. A woman wants to use the calendar method of fertility control. She keeps a record of her menstrual cycle for 12 months. Her shortest cycle is 26 days. Her longest cycle is 33 days. What are fertile days in her cycle? What days should she abstain from penis-vagina contact in order to avoid pregnancy?

____

____

____

____

____

2. Suppose you or your spouse just found out that you are expecting a child in eight months. Identify concerns for prenatal care that you would have.

____

____

____

____

____

3. Jenny just found out that she is six weeks pregnant. This is her first pregnancy and she does not know what to expect. Describe the changes that will occur during each trimester of her pregnancy.

____

____

____

____

____

4. Aiko is expecting a baby in two months. She learns that the American Academy of Pediatrics has strongly recommended that full-term newborns be breast-fed. What are the advantages of breast-feeding? When deciding whether to breast- or bottle-feed, what should she consider?

5. Rashida is expecting her second child in 6 months. For her first child, she experienced a traditional hospital birth and was dissatisfied. What are her options for her second infant's birth and her participation in it?

Critical Thinking Activity: The Possibility of Parenthood

If you are sexually active, there is a chance that you or your partner could become pregnant. Choosing if and when to have children is a great responsibility. A woman and her partner have much to consider before planning or risking a pregnancy. Before you plan or risk a pregnancy, you have the responsibility to make certain you are physically, emotionally, and financially prepared to care for another human being. Assume you are about to become a parent and answer the following questions based upon this assumption.

1. Why do you want to have a child?

2. How will you financially provide for your child?

3. Will both you and your partner work or will one of you stay home with the child?

4. What health behaviors will you change for the sake of the unborn child?

5. What birth method will you choose? Why?

6. Who will you turn to for answers on how to raise your child?

7. Will you need additional space in your home?

8. What parenting skills do you possess?

9. How much experience do you have raising children?

10. How will you provide for the child should something happen to you and your partner?

Language Enrichment Glossary

In addition to the words in the Key Terms list at the end of the chapter, students listed the following words as difficult to understand. Use the Key Terms list, this list, your dictionary, and teachers and friends to learn the meaning of words you do not understand.

adage:	saying
affords:	gives, allows
ascertain:	determine
at risk for:	in danger of
attributable to:	caused by
barrier:	a block
burrows:	buries or digs itself into
calculated:	figured
cervical:	related to the opening of the uterus
chronic:	lasting, repeated, persistent
clots:	thickened lumps of blood
complications:	related problems
comprehensive:	broad, including many things
compromising:	risky
conducive:	favorable
conscientious:	careful
constitute:	make up
contractions:	muscle squeezing
conventional:	customary, standard
debilitating:	weakening
depletion:	lowering
differentiates:	separates
discernible:	understandable, discoverable
disintegrate:	break apart, decay
dislodged:	moved out of place
emits:	sends out
ensure:	guarantee
entail:	involve, require
hemorrhage:	bleeding which doesn't stop
impose:	place, force
in conjunction with:	together with
inflammatory:	becoming red, swollen and painful
intramuscularly:	into the muscle
lesions:	open wounds
metabolizes:	how a substance acts in the body
misshapen:	shaped incorrectly
readily:	easily
render:	result in, cause to be
reversible:	able to change back to original
revert:	go back to, return
shunning:	avoiding
sluggish:	slow
spontaneity:	happening without planning
stump:	short end still left after being cut
subsequent:	following
succumbing:	giving in

suffice:	be enough
suppresses:	stops
synthetic:	artificial, human-made
transfusion:	adding blood to the bloodstream
undue:	too much, excessive
viable:	living

CHAPTER 9

ADDICTIONS AND ADDICTIVE BEHAVIOR: THREATS TO WELLNESS

Chapter Overview

Addiction is defined as continued involvement with a substance or activity despite ongoing negative consequences. All addictions are characterized by compulsion, loss of control, negative consequences, and denial.

Addiction is a process that evolves over time. The progression of addiction can be understood on an emotional continuum. Vernon E. Johnson's Feeling Chart illustrates the five-phase process an addict goes through on an emotional level: learning the mood swing, seeking the mood swing, harmful dependency, using to feel normal, and harmful dependency again. Mood-altering substances and experiences produce tolerance and withdrawal. The most effective treatment today relies on the biopsychosocial model to explain addiction. According to this model, addiction is caused by a variety of factors, including biological and sociocultural influences, life events, and family influences.

"Process addictions" are behaviors known to be addictive because they are mood-altering. Money addictions include compulsive gambling and compulsive shopping. A work addiction is the compulsive use of work and the work persona to fulfill needs of intimacy, power, and success. Addictive exercisers use compulsive exercise to try to meet needs that cannot be met by any object or activity, such as nurturing, intimacy, and self-esteem. Sex addicts compulsively seek sexual arousal and are often indifferent about who or what activity provides it. Most addicts are dependent on more than one chemical and/or behavior, even though they tend to have a "drug of choice" or a "behavior of choice."

Recognition is one of the most difficult steps in the process of recovery due to the addict's denial. Intervention is a planned process of confrontation by significant others. Its purpose is to break down the denial compassionately so that the addict can see the destructive nature of the addiction. Once recognition has been achieved, recovery can begin. Treatment and recovery for any addiction begins with abstinence. Abstinence means refraining from the addictive behavior, while detoxification refers to the early abstinence period in which an addict adjusts physically and cognitively to being free from the influence of the addiction. But abstinence is not enough. Successful treatment also requires recovery, a new way of looking at oneself, others, and the world. Recovery programs are necessary for addicts to resist relapsing. For many addicts, recovery begins with a period of formal treatment. Most programs use a combination of family, individual, and group counseling supplemented with attendance at a 12-step support group. Relapse is one of the defining characteristics of addiction. Because treatment programs recognize this strong tendency to return to addictive behavior, they routinely teach concepts of relapse prevention. Women in need of recovery from addictions often have barriers at the individual, family, and societal levels. Treatment centers need to overcome gender-based treatment barriers.

Learning Objectives

1. Distinguish addictions from habits and identify the signs of addiction.

2. Discuss the addictive process, the physiology of addiction, and the biopsychosocial model of addiction.

3. Describe the types of addictions, including money addictions, work addiction, exercise addiction, sexual addictions, and codependence.

4. Evaluate treatment and recovery for addicts, including individual therapy, group therapy, family therapy, and 12-step programs.

Key Terms

Fill in a brief definition to help you remember these terms.

addiction ______

withdrawal ______

relapse ______

habit ______

compulsion ______

obsession ______

loss of control ______

negative consequences ______

denial ______

nurturing through avoidance ______

neurotransmitters ______

tolerance ______

biopsychosocial model of addiction ______

social learning theory ______

enablers ______

compulsive gambler ______

work addiction ______

addictive exercisers ______

codependence ______

intervention ______

abstinence ______

detoxification ______

Short Answers

1. In order for a behavior to be addictive, what potential must a behavior have?

cause pos. mood change

2. What is the difference between a habit and an addiction.

habit can be controlled

3. Identify four components that are present in all addictions.

(1) compulsion
(2) loss of control
(3) neg. consequence
(4) denial

4. What are the five phases of addiction?

(1) learns mood swing
(2) seeks mood swing
(3) harmful dependancy to feel high
(4) drinks/shoots to be normal
(5) harmful dependance to feel normal

5. Explain the phenomena of tolerance and withdrawal associated with mood-altering experiences.

tolerance – larger doses needed
withdrawl – to feel normal

6. What are key risk factors for addictions?

Biological – alcol in parents, life events, disease family influences.

7. What is codependence?

addicted to the addict

8. What does treatment and recovery for any addiction begin with?

abstinance

9. What is the purpose of an intervention?

To make person break denial

10. What is a relapse?

going back to addiction

Critical Thinking Exercises

1. In family therapy for compulsive gambling, Nathan's therapist listens to his parents explain how they have loaned him money on numerous occasions and paid Nathan's rent whenever he lost it through gambling. How do Nathan's parents enable him to continue the addiction?

2. Describe the profile of a 40-year-old man suffering from work addiction.

3. Jane is an addictive exerciser. In what way does she abuse exercise? What negative consequences result from her addiction?

4. A social worker from an addiction treatment center has agreed to meet with a family who has requested an intervention for their alcoholic father. What skills would help them have an effective confrontation?

5. Suppose you are a consultant for gender issues in addiction treatment centers. You have been asked to discuss obstacles that may affect whether or not women receive the help they need. What do you tell the staff?

Critical Thinking Activity: Treatment and Recovery for Addiction

Suppose you have just been named the director of an addiction treatment center. What would be the major components of your program? What should your facility provide clients to ensure a good treatment program? Who would be key staff members? What expectations would you have for your staff? What strategies would you use for overcoming gender-based treatment barriers? What would be the mission statement of your treatment center, reflecting your philosophy about treatment expectations?

Language Enrichment Glossary

In addition to the words in the Key Terms list at the end of the chapter, students listed the following words as difficult to understand. Use the chapter Key Terms list, this list, your dictionary, and teachers and friends to learn th meaning of words you do not understand.

barbiturate:	a sedative drug
compulsive eating:	emotional need to eat often or too much
constricted:	squeezed
cordial:	friendly, polite

critically:	significantly
cross-dressing:	emotional pleasure in dressing as the opposite sex
discord:	conflict, disagreement
disintegration:	deterioration, breaking apart
dissolution:	dissolving, breaking apart
enhancer:	intensifier, increaser
euphoric:	a feeling of great happiness
falsification:	misrepresenting, lying
gastrointestinal tract:	digestive system
idolized celebrities:	admired famous people
incest:	sexual intercourse with a close blood relative
incur:	acquire
insidious:	hidden danger
integrate:	include
manipulative:	attempt to dominate, control another
martini:	type of alcoholic cocktail drink
moderate:	control
mood-altering:	changes emotional states
naive:	foolish, uninformed
notion:	idea
orgasm:	climax from sexual excitement
pedophilia:	adult sexual activity with a child
peer-led:	led by people equal to those following
perfectionist:	person with too-high standards
pervasive:	widespread
phenomenon:	occurrence, event
prime time:	most-watched evening television period
profound:	strong, deep
promiscuous:	having many casual sexual partners
repetitious:	done over and over
riddled with:	filled with
spiritually-based:	set on religious beliefs
stigma:	mark of social shame
subordinate:	suppress, make less important
tranquilizers:	mood-calming drugs
voyeurism:	sexual pleasure from secretly observing another

CHAPTER 10
PHARMACEUTICAL DRUGS: SAFE AND RESPONSIBLE USE

Chapter Overview

Drugs work because they physically resemble the chemicals produced naturally within the body. Scientists divide drugs into six categories: prescription drugs, over-the-counter preparations, recreational substances, herbal preparations, illicit drugs, and commercial drugs. The way in which a given drug is taken into the body is called the route of administration. Common routes are oral ingestion, injection, inhalation, inunction, and suppository.

The use of a drug for a purpose for which it was not intended is called drug misuse. Drug abuse is the excessive use of any drug. The misuse and abuse of drugs may lead to addiction. Creating a drug profile before you decide whether to use a chemical substance can help you intelligently weigh the risks and benefits of a particular drug. Individuals respond differently to psychoactive drugs. Two environmental factors that bear on both the main effects and the side effects of psychoactive drugs are set and setting. Set is the total internal environment, or mindset, of a person at the time a drug is taken, while the setting refers to the external environment of a person at the time a drug is taken. Polydrug use, or taking several medications or illegal drugs simultaneously, may cause very dangerous problems associated with drug interactions. The most hazardous interactions are synergism, antagonism, inhibition, and intolerance.

Prescription drugs are administered under medical supervision. Types of prescription drugs include antibiotics, analgesics, sedatives, tranquilizers, antidepressants, and amphetamines. Generic drugs are medications sold under their chemical name and contain the same active ingredient as their brand-name counterparts. Even though generic drugs are often less expensive than their brand-name counterparts, not all drugs are available as generics, and generic equivalents are not always recommended.

Over-the-counter (OTC) drugs are those nonprescription drugs we use in the course of self-diagnosis and self-medication. In response to consumer pressures, the Food and Drug Administration (FDA) has adopted a switching policy whereby it regularly reviews prescription drugs to evaluate how suitable they would be as OTC products. The most commonly used over-the-counter drugs are analgesics, cold/cough/allergy and asthma relievers, stimulants, sleeping aids and relaxants, and dieting aids. Consumers should exercise personal responsibility by reading directions for OTC drugs and asking their pharmacist or doctor if any special precautions are advised when taking these drugs.

Learning Objectives

1. List the six categories of drugs and explain the routes of administration that drugs take into the body.

2. Discuss proper drug use and explain how hazardous drug interactions occur.

3. Describe the various kinds of prescription drugs and the advantages that generic drugs may provide to consumers.

4. Discuss the types of over-the-counter drugs and general precautions to be taken when using them.

5. Explain why people are concerned about the FDA's lack of monitoring of herbal products.

Key Terms

Fill in a brief definition to help you remember these terms.

227 receptor sites Specialized cells where drugs attach

227 psychoactive drugs drugs that alter mood or behavior

227 prescription drugs Medications that have prescrip

227 over-the-counter (OTC) drugs Med. w/o prescrip

229 recreational drugs contain chemicals that help to relax

herbal preparations substances originate from plants

illicit (illegal) drugs illegal drugs that cause harm,

commercial preparations commonly used house products

route of administration manner drug is taken

oral ingestion Taking drug through mouth

injection " " with needle

intravenous injection " " in vein

intramuscular injection " " in muscles

subcutaneous injection " " in fat

inhalation " " through mouth/nose

inunction introduced through skin

suppositories per rectum or vagina

drug misuse drug use for unintended reason

229 drug abuse " " excessively

231 set mind set at time drug taken

231 setting external environment person takes

231 polydrug use

233 synergism interaction of 2 or more drugs to make more po

233 antagonism 2 more drugs work same site where one block the other

inhibition ____________________

intolerance ____________________

cross-tolerance ____________________

antibiotics ____________________

analgesics ____________________

prostaglandin inhibitors ____________________

sedatives ____________________

tranquilizers ____________________

antidepressants ____________________

amphetamines ____________________

rebound effects ____________________

generic drugs ____________________

GRAS list ____________________

GRAE list ____________________

sympathomimetics ____________________

laxative ____________________

diuretic ____________________

Short Answers

1. A current explanation of drug actions is the receptor site theory. Explain the receptor site theory.

2. List three examples of a recreational drug.

3. Name the five common routes of administration of drugs.

oral iv
rectal inhalation

4. What is the difference between drug misuse and drug abuse?

5. One environmental factor that bears on both the main effects and side effects of psychoactive drugs is "setting." Define setting in this context.

6. Define synergism. When is a synergistic interaction most likely to occur?

7. What is Antabuse and how does it work?

8. What are antibiotics used for?

9. Define "over-the-counter" drugs.

10. How do prescription drugs become over-the-counter drugs?

11. What are possible side effects of aspirin use?

12. How do expectorants work?

Critical Thinking Exercises

1. Lyle, your friend from high school, is staying with you while going through a divorce. He likes to drink alcohol, and now you see that he has prescription barbiturates to help him sleep. What concern do you have about Lyle mixing alcohol and barbiturates?

2. Ann takes ibuprofen, a prostaglandin inhibitor, for her menstrual cramps. How does this drug work?

3. Jody has been seeing a doctor due to her anxiety attacks. The doctor has been prescribing Valium for over two years. Should she have any reason for concern? Why or why not?

4. Your friend, Kayla, has been using prescription amphetamines for several months to treat obesity.. Now she is ready to quit. What rebound effects might she experience?

5. Your friend is sick and asks you to pick up her prescription drugs at the pharmacy. She asks your advice about using a generic form of the drug. What do you tell her?

6. Your friend, Laura, has been using laxatives and diuretics to lose weight and she brags that she has lost two dress sizes, seeking your approval. What do you say to her about the health consequences of her actions?

7. Tom is moving away from home to attend college. His parents are concerned about his health knowledge, and they want him to be informed about over-the-counter medications. What are some guidelines for safe self-treatment?

____

____

____

____

____

Critical Thinking Activity: Your Safe and Responsible Use of Prescription Drugs

Visiting a physician does not exempt you from exercising responsibility for your own health. Too often, individuals simply take the prescription medication without asking basic questions about the medication and just assume that the doctor knows best. Answer the following questions about your pattern of prescription drug use.

1. I take prescription drugs.

   Always Usually Sometimes Rarely Never

2. I ask questions about why I am being given a specific prescription.

   Always Usually Sometimes Rarely Never

3. I inform the doctor or pharmacist of any allergies to medications.

   Always Usually Sometimes Rarely Never

4. I know the side effects of the prescription drugs that I take.

   Always Usually Sometimes Rarely Never

5. I know the benefits of the prescription drugs I take.

   Always Usually Sometimes Rarely Never

6. I know how my prescription drug should be administered.

   Always Usually Sometimes Rarely Never

7. I know whether my prescription drug is available as a generic drug.

   Always Usually Sometimes Rarely Never

8. I have accepted my doctor's recommendation regarding medication.

   Always Usually Sometimes Rarely Never

9. I take my prescription drug as instructed.

   Always Usually Sometimes Rarely Never

Questions for the Critical Thinker

After you have completed this exercise, reflect on the following questions. Your thoughtful responses will enhance your learning of this activity as well as your knowledge of pharmaceutical drugs.

1. What do your answers suggest about how good a consumer you are when it comes to medication?

2. How much responsibility have you assumed for your use of prescription drugs?

3. What do you need to improve, if anything?

4. Do you think your level of consumerism is typical?

Language Enrichment Glossary

In addition to the words in the Key Terms list at the end of the chapter, students listed the following words as difficult to understand. Use the chapter Key Terms list, this list, your dictionary, and teachers and friends to learn the meaning of words you do not understand.

adhesive patches:	sticky skin pad containing chemicals
ails:	troubles, disturbs
alleviate:	reduce, soothe
anesthetics:	painkillers
antacid:	product reducing stomach acid pain
benign:	good or harmless
compile:	gather, collect
complement:	addition to
constipation:	difficulty moving bowels
controversy:	disagreement, conflict
corrosive:	causes erosion or deterioration
cultivation:	encourage to grow, develop
curtail:	limit, reduce
depletion:	reduction of, loss of
derivatives:	something that came from something else
diminish:	reduce

dispensed:	distributed
dispersion:	spread throughout
disrupts:	disturbs, interrupts
fatigue:	tiredness
fetus:	unborn baby
giddy:	dizzy, silly
hallucinations:	imagined visions which seem real
hypodermic syringe:	needle and plunger to inject something
ingrown nails:	nails which grow painfully into the skin
metabolized:	chemical process of absorbing
nauseated:	stomach upset
neglected:	not paid attention to
notorious:	negatively well-known
obligations:	commitments, responsibilities
opium poppy:	flower containing opium
physiology:	biological process
possess:	have, contain
prescribed:	recommended by a doctor
prevails:	succeeds
remedies:	treatments
sanctioned:	approved
unforeseeable:	unexpected
unspectacular:	not outstanding, unsuccessful
waxy medium:	wax used to mix with something

CHAPTER 11
DRINKING RESPONSIBLY: A LIFESTYLE CHALLENGE

Chapter Overview

As a society, we refuse to categorize alcohol as a drug because it is socially accepted. But you should remember that alcohol is a chemical substance that affects your physical and mental behavior. The drinking of alcohol is interwoven with our traditions. An estimated 7 out of 10 Americans consume alcoholic beverages regularly. Alcohol is the most widely used recreational drug in our society, and is the most popular drug on college campuses, where 85 percent of students consume alcoholic beverages. About 25 percent abuse alcohol. Binge drinking on college campuses has become a big problem. Although everyone is at some risk for alcoholism and alcohol-related problems, college students seem to be particularly vulnerable. Many colleges and universities are making efforts to prevent alcohol abuse. A decrease in per capita alcohol consumption occurred between 1981 and 1995.

Behavioral changes caused by alcohol vary with the set and setting and with the individual. Blood alcohol concentration is used to measure the physiological and behavioral effects of alcohol. How quickly the body absorbs alcohol is influenced by several factors, including the alcohol concentration in the drink, the amount of alcohol consumed, the amount of food in your stomach, and your mood. A drinker's blood alcohol content also depends on weight and body fat, the water content in body tissues, the rate of consumption, and the volume of alcohol consumed. Women have half as much of the enzyme that breaks down alcohol in the stomach. Therefore if a man and a woman both drink the same amount of alcohol, the woman's blood alcohol content will be 30 percent higher than the man's. The most dramatic immediate effects produced by alcohol occur in the central nervous system, leading to decreases in respiratory rate, pulse rate, and blood pressure. In extreme cases, coma and death can result. A hangover is often experienced the morning after a drinking spree. Chronic alcohol consumption can have serious cumulative effects, including effects on the nervous system, cardiovascular effects, liver disease, and cancer. Fetal alcohol syndrome is associated with alcohol consumption throughout pregnancy. Approximately 41 percent of all traffic fatalities are alcohol-related.

Alcohol use turns into alcohol abuse or alcoholism when it interferes with work, school, social or family relationships, or when it entails any violation of the law. Ninety-five percent of alcoholics live in some type of extended family unit. They can be found at all levels of society. Women are the fastest-growing component of the population of alcohol abusers. Alcohol is a disease with biological, psychological, and social/environmental components. A family history of alcoholism may predispose a person to problems with alcohol. Certain social factors have been linked to alcoholism, including urbanization, the weakening of links to the extended family, increased mobility, and changing religious and philosophical values. The alcoholic's entire family suffers from the disease of alcoholism. An estimated 30 million Americans come from an alcoholic household. The entire society also suffers the consequences of individuals' alcohol abuse. The annual cost of alcohol-related crimes, medical expenses, accidents, and treatment programs is about $100 billion.

Less than 10 percent of alcoholics in the United States receive any care. An intervention is an effective method of helping an alcoholic to confront the disease. An alcoholic can get treatment from private treatment facilities, family therapy, individual therapy, group therapy, drug and aversion therapy, or Alcoholics Anonymous and other self-help groups. Roughly 60 percent of alcoholics relapse within the first three months of treatment. Alcoholics most likely to recover completely are those who developed their dependencies after the age of 20, those with intact and supportive family units, and those who have reached a high level of personal disgust coupled with strong motivation to recover.

Learning Objectives

1. Summarize the alcohol use patterns of college students and discuss overall trends in consumption.

2. Explain the physiological and behavioral effects of alcohol, including blood alcohol concentration, absorption, metabolism, and immediate and long-term effects of alcohol consumption.

3. Explain the symptoms and causes of alcoholism, its cost to society, and its effects on the family.

4. Explain the treatment of alcoholism, including the family's role, varied treatment methods, and whether or not alcoholics can be cured.

Key Terms

Fill in a brief definition to help you remember these terms.

binge drinking drinking too much at one time

ethyl alcohol (ethanol) fancy word for alcohol

fermentation process of yeast to alcy

distillation process of high temp release of sugar

proof % of alcohol

blood-alcohol concentration (BAC) ratio of Alcohol : Blood

learned behavioral tolerance ability not to look drunk when you are

dehydration loss of bodily tissues

cerebrospinal fluid fluid around spinal cord

hangover bad morning diarea anxiety

congeners what is left over in alcohol that cause hangover

cirrhosis last stage of liver cancer

alcohol hepatitis inflamed liver from too much drink

fetal alcohol syndrome (FAS) disorder caused from moms drink

fetal alcohol effects (FAE) affects of FAS

alcohol abuse (alcoholism) use of alcohol that affects school, life

intervention planned confrontation

delirium tremens (DTs) state of confusion from withdraw

Alcoholics Anonymous Organization to stop drinking

Short Answers

1. What are the negative effects of alcohol use on student behavior?

Date Rape, STD

2. What is used to measure the physiological and behavioral effects of alcohol?

Blood A/C Conc
(BAC)

3. What factors affect how quickly your system will absorb alcohol?

fat amount in body
food in body / male/female

4. If a man and a woman both drink the same amount of alcohol, why is the woman's blood-alcohol concentration about 30 percent higher than the man's?

Body fat
1/2 hydrogenous

5. What are the effects of fetal alcohol syndrome?

FAS wide eyes, low ears

6. Distinguish between Type 1 and Type 2 alcoholism.

...type 1 raised in alcy environ
...gical " 2 ~~born~~ born to alcoholic parents

7. What social factors have been linked with alcoholism?

difficulties forming relations,
family prob, wedding

8. Cite differences between men and women when it comes to alcohol abuse.

men to get drunk/Bond
women to social

9. How does Antabuse work in the treatment of alcoholism?

Makes them sick

10. What is the purpose of Alateen?

AA for teenagers

11. What is the relapse rate for alcoholics within the first three months of treatment?

60%

12. Which alcoholics are most likely to recover completely?

those who start drinking after the age of 20

Critical Thinking Exercises

1. What are your college policies related to alcohol consumption? What help is available to students with drinking problems? What efforts are directed toward the prevention of alcohol abuse?

_____

_____

_____

_____

_____

2. Suppose you are having a New Year's Eve party for a group of friends. What are some actions you can take to ensure that your guests drink responsibly?

_____

_____

_____

_____

3. Suppose you have been asked to present a lecture on the long-term effects of alcohol consumption to patients in a treatment recovery program. What long-term effects would you address?

4. Nancy lives in a dysfunctional family. Her father is an alcoholic and compulsive gambler. Nancy diverts attention away from her father by refusing to eat at family meals, exercising excessively, and losing a significant amount of weight. Nancy's anorexic behaviors may be the result of assuming what role in her family?

5. Jonah is an alcoholic. After an intervention involving his family members and a therapist, he has agreed to enter a treatment program.. When he does quit drinking, what withdrawal symptoms is he most likely to experience?

Critical Thinking Activity: Alcohol Advertising Appeal

Using newspapers and magazines, find an example of each of the following:

A beer or a liquor ad that portrays alcohol consumption as

*a healthy activity

*an activity of the wealthy

*a fun activity

*sexually arousing

*masculine

*feminine

*patriotic

*a health risk

*a dangerous activity to be undertaken with caution

Next, design an advertisement that addresses one consequence of alcohol abuse on society. The advertisement should arouse consumer interest and at the same time rely on factual information rather than shallow imagery. Use the space below to create your advertisement.

Questions for the Critical Thinker

After you have found the advertisements and created one of your own, reflect on the following questions. Your thoughtful responses will enhance your learning of this activity as well as your understanding of drinking responsibly.

1. Based on your review of the above advertisements, do you think alcohol advertisements should be more closely regulated? Why or why not?

2. Can you think of an alcohol advertisement that has appealed to you? What made it persuasive?

3. How could the information in your advertisement be useful in a college setting?

4. What is an effective way to reach out to college students with a drinking problem?

Language Enrichment Glossary

In addition to the words in the Key Terms list at the end of the chapter, students listed the following words as difficult to understand. Use the Key Terms list, this list, your dictionary, and teachers and friends to learn the meaning of words you do not understand.

abstinence:	not do something
abysmal:	extremely bad
access:	reach, obtain
acquaintance rape:	forced sex by known person
adapt:	adjust
adhere:	follow, stick to
adjunct:	addition, supplement
affliction:	illness, problem
agitated:	disturbed, excited
alert:	warn, notify
antagonizing:	offending, annoying
auxiliary group:	group connected to a main group
aversive properties:	offensive characteristics
blatant:	obvious, stand out

bombarded:	attacked, overwhelmed
causative factor:	a cause of something
coma:	long, deep unconsciousness
component:	part
comprehensive:	broad, complete
compulsive:	addicted
concentration:	amount of something present
concerted:	focused on one thing
condones:	allows, permits
confronts:	challenges
converted:	changed
decisive:	definite, determining
delusions:	false perceptions
dependent on:	need or rely on something
designate:	choose
diffuse:	spread out
dilute:	weaken
dominated:	controlled
doomed:	expected bad outcome
drinking spree:	overindulgence in drinking
dump:	toss out, unload
endured:	suffered, tolerated
enhance:	intensify
entails:	involves
eradicate:	eliminate, get rid of
err on the side of:	make a cautious, conservative choice
euphoric:	feeling of great happiness
exacerbate:	make worse
excreted:	eliminated from, pushed out of
exert:	creates
extended family:	relatives beyond immediate family
fibrous:	resembling fibers twisted together
gauging:	measuring
higher power:	spiritual belief in something greater than humans
impinge upon:	influence negatively
in conjunction with:	happens at the same time
inalienable right:	undeniable, absolute right
inconclusive:	indefinite, undetermined
indication:	measure
inebriated:	drunk
inhibit:	slow down, restrict
inhibitions:	personal reservations
instituting:	establishing
interfere:	interrupt, obstruct
intoxicated:	drunk
judiciously:	choose carefully
liqueurs:	sweet, condensed alcoholic drinks
localized:	staying in a specific area
loosen up:	relax
metabolized:	physical process of being absorbed into the body
moderate:	reasonable, not extreme

monitor:	watch, supervise
motor impairment:	muscle handicap
negligible:	unimportant, insignificant
noxious:	unpleasant, repulsive
optional complement:	voluntary addition
over-attend:	pay too much attention
overrepresented:	more than expected
peers:	equals
per capita:	per person
perpetuate:	help to continue
predispose:	tendency toward
primarily:	mainly, basically
prioritized:	placed in order of importance
prolonged:	continued, extended
readily:	easily, quickly
receptor:	nerve ending which receives a stimulus
recreational drug:	drug taken for pleasure
refrain:	avoid doing something
resiliency:	ability to bounce back from problems
resolve:	decide, commit
retards:	slows
revocation:	cancellation
setting:	surrounding situation
shrinkage:	contraction, becoming smaller
sobering:	serious, solemn
social living group:	people in one's daily life
stigma:	social disgrace, shame
solution:	mixture
spouse battering:	physical abuse of spouse
steadfastly:	unfailingly
suffocate:	die from lack of air in lungs
synaptic junctions:	points of nerve connections
tolerance to:	resistance to
transported:	carried
trend:	tendency
unwitting:	unaware
urbanization:	becoming like a city
value-related:	connected with morals and beliefs
variable:	various, changeable
vital functions:	temperature, pulse and breathing rate
vulnerable:	sensitive to something

CHAPTER 12

TOBACCO AND CAFFEINE: LEGAL ADDICTIONS

Chapter Overview

The single most preventable cause of death in the United States is the use of tobacco. One in every five deaths in the United States is smoking-related.

Tobacco is sold in several forms: cigarettes, cigars, pipes, snuff, and chewing tobacco. The chemical stimulant nicotine is the major psychoactive substance in all these tobacco products. Nicotine is a powerful central nervous system stimulant that causes a variety of physiological effects. Its stimulant action in the cerebral cortex produces an aroused, alert mental state. Nicotine also stimulates the adrenal glands, increasing the production of adrenaline. The physical effects of nicotine stimulation include increased heart and respiratory rate, constriction of blood vessels, and subsequent increased blood pressure. Nicotine decreases the stomach contractions that signal hunger, decreases blood sugar levels, and decreases the sensation in the taste buds.

Tobacco smoking has been directly linked to cancer, cardiovascular disease, respiratory disorders, and gum disease. Female smokers have a greater risk of developing cervical cancer and heart disease than do female nonsmokers. Smoking also appears to cause women to begin menopause prematurely and contributes to osteoporosis. Cigarette smoking presents special dangers for pregnant women and their fetuses, including miscarriages, low birthweights, higher infant mortality rates, and higher rates of sudden infant death syndrome.

Smokeless tobacco is used by approximately 5 million Americans. There are two types of smokeless tobacco--chewing tobacco and snuff. Smokeless tobacco is just as addictive as cigarettes due to its nicotine content. In fact, smokeless tobacco has more nicotine than cigarettes. One of the major risks of chewing tobacco is leukoplakia, and between 3 and 17 percent of diagnosed leukoplakia cases develop into oral cancer.

Environmental tobacco smoke is divided into two categories: mainstream smoke and sidestream smoke. Approximately 9 out of 10 nonsmoking Americans are exposed to environmental tobacco smoke. Involuntary smokers face risks from exposure to tobacco smoke because secondhand smoke actually contains more carcinogenic substances than the smoke that a smoker inhales. In fact, the Environmental Protection Agency has designated secondhand tobacco smoke a group A cancer-causing agent and has also concluded that secondhand smoke increases the risk of pneumonia and bronchitis in children.

Quitting smoking is difficult. There are a variety of methods to help the smoker quit, including quitting "cold turkey", nicotine chewing gum, the nicotine patch, the nicotine nasal spray, aversion therapy, operant conditioning, and self-control therapy. There are numerous health benefits of quitting smoking. For instance, at the end of 10 smoke-free years, the ex-smoker can expect to live out his or her normal life span.

Caffeine is a drug derived from the chemical family called xanthines, which are mild central nervous system stimulants that enhance mental alertness and reduce fatigue. Side effects of xanthines include wakefulness, insomnia, irregular heartbeat, dizziness, nausea, indigestion, and sometimes mild delirium. Caffeinism is caffeine intoxication caused by excessive caffeine use, with symptoms including chronic insomnia, jitters, irritability, nervousness, anxiety, and involuntary muscle twitches. Moderate caffeine consumption produces very few harmful effects in healthy, nonpregnant people.

Learning Objectives

1. Discuss the social issues involved in tobacco use, including advertising and the medical costs associated with tobacco use.

2. Discuss how the chemicals in tobacco products affect a smoker's body.

3. Review how smoking affects a smoker's risk for cancer, cardiovascular disease, and respiratory diseases, and how it adversely affects a fetus's health.

4. Discuss the risks associated with using smokeless tobacco.

5. Evaluate the risks to nonsmokers associated with environmental tobacco smoke.

6. Describe strategies people adopt to quit using tobacco products, including strategies aimed at breaking the nicotine addiction as well as the habit.

7. Compare the benefits and risks associated with caffeine, and summarize the health consequences of long-term caffeine use.

Key Terms

Fill in a brief definition to help you remember these terms.

snuff ____________________

chewing tobacco ____________________

nicotine ____________________

tar ____________________

carbon monoxide ____________________

nicotine poisoning ____________________

platelet adhesiveness ____________________

emphysema ____________________

sudden infant death syndrome (SIDS) ____________________

leukoplakia ____________________

environmental tobacco smoke (ETS) ____________________

mainstream smoke ____________________

sidestream smoke ____________________

nicotine withdrawal Stop smoking (nausea/headache)

caffeine Stimulant (coffee/soda/tea/chocolate)

xanthines family of stimulates (caffeine family)

caffeinism intoxification of excessive caffeine use.

Short Answers

1. What are the physiological effects of nicotine?

stimulates action in cerebral cortex, aroused alert mental state, stimulate adrenal glands.

2. How does smoking contribute to heart disease?

adding 10 years to aging of arteries. Lowers HDL

3. What physical problems are female smokers at risk for?

cervical cancer and heart disease higher risk Breast lung cancer

4. Besides cancer, what are the health risks created by smokeless tobacco?

leukoplakia. leathery patches in mouth

5. What are the pro and con arguments concerning the use of nicotine replacement gum?

contains nicotine, substitutes one addiction for another, experience no withdrawal and fewer cravings for nicotine.

6. How does the nicotine patch work?

placed on upper body, delivers cont. flow of nicotines through the skin

7. List health benefits of quitting smoking.

Live longer
smokers breath disappears
no yellow teeth
less chance of cancer
save money

8. What are the symptoms of caffeinism?

headache
chronic insomnia
irritability
anxiety muscle twiches

Critical Thinking Exercises

1. Angie is a good friend of yours, but she adamantly refuses to give up smoking. Whenever you raise the subject, she answers, "What do you care? It's not like you pay for my habit." How does smoking hurt nonsmokers financially?

____

____

____

____

____

2. Your friend, Edna, finally listens to your warnings about the dangers of tobacco smoking. She tells you that after giving it much thought, she is switching to clove cigarettes. What is your reaction?

____

____

____

____

____

3. Cindy and Liz are best friends, but Cindy's smoking really bothers Liz. When Liz asks Cindy not to smoke when they are together, Cindy says, "I'm only hurting myself, not you." Is she correct? Why or why not?

____

____

____

____

____

4. Bill has smoked a pack of cigarettes a day for the past eight years. He wants to quit smoking, but thinks that he has already caused damage to his body, so he doesn't see any reason to quit now. What are the benefits of quitting?

____

____

____

____

____

5. Your mother has been a very heavy coffee drinker for several years. Now she has reduced her consumption and is a moderate coffee drinker. Your father insists that she cut out all coffee and says that there is no acceptable level of coffee consumption. What does the data say about the effects of moderate caffeine use?

____

____

____

____

____

Critical Thinking Activity

Billboards are no longer allowed for tobacco advertising. In fact, anti-smoking billboards are springing up all across America. In the space below, create your own anti-smoking billboard to deter tobacco use.

Questions for the Critical Thinker

After you have completed your billboard, reflect on the following questions. Your thoughtful responses will enhance your learning of this activity as well as your understanding of psychosocial health.

1. What groups should anti-smoking billboards target?

Teens + young adults

2. What legislative controls, if any, should be used to regulate tobacco smoke?

Raises age to 21

3. Are you satisfied with current legislation regarding secondhand smoke?

yes it could be better though.

Language Enrichment Glossary

In addition to the words in the Key Terms list at the end of the chapter, students listed the following words as difficult to understand. Use the chapter Key Terms list, this list, your dictionary, and teachers and friends to learn the meaning of words you do not understand.

abnormality:	something wrong
absorbed:	soaked in
accumulate:	gather
achieved:	accomplished
addictive:	creating a need
adolescents:	teenagers
adversely:	negatively
airways:	breathing passages
analyzed:	studied, examined
appetite:	desire to eat
aroused:	stimulated
arteries:	large blood vessels
attaining:	reaching
banned:	prevented, eliminated
bloodstream:	blood
bowling alley:	place to do bowling game
buildup:	increase, gathering
bus depot:	bus station
cannot stand:	strongly dislike
carcinogenic:	causes cancer
cardiac patient:	heart patient
cardiovascular:	related to heart and blood circulation

cerebral cortex: part of the brain
cessation: stopping
characteristics: qualities
chewers: people who chew tobacco
chronic: constant, frequent
cigarette-induced: caused by smoking
circulatory: blood system
clogging: blocking, plugging up
clotting: lumps of blood
compensate: to make up for
comprehensive: broad, includes many things
constantly: without stopping
consumed: to drink or eat
continuously: without stopping
contraceptives: birth control
contractions: squeezing
correlated: associated
counseling: talking treatment
cravings: desires for something
culprit: negative cause
cure: remedy to heal a disease
decaffeinated: caffeine taken out
deformities: unhealthy development
denying: preventing
depicted: shown
depleted: lowered
deprivation: shortage
derive: gain, obtain from
despite: in spite of
diagnosed: identified
diminish: make smaller
dippers: people who suck tobacco
disputed: argued about
distribution: to deliver, spread
domestic: within a country
dosage: amount
dramatically: significantly
eliminate: get rid of, take away
emphysema: lung disease
emulating: imitating
enacted: made
enhance: increase
enlarged: made bigger
entice: tempt
exhale: breathe out
exhausted: very tired
expelled: sent out
extraordinary: unusual
extremely: very

fast food: already prepared food
fatal: causes death
fatigue: tiredness
fetuses: unborn babies not completely formed
flawed: containing mistakes
graduate: to move on to
habit: customary behavior
harmless: doesn't damage
hazardous: dangerous
heartbeat: pulses of the heart
heartburn: stomach indigestion
impairs: limits
in contrast: in comparison
ingest: drink or eat
inhaling: breathing smoke into the lungs
insomnia: inability to sleep
intensive: deep, strong
irritants: things which bother, inflame
irritate: bother, inflame
jawbone: bone in bottom of face
lag: delay
letdown: tired, sad feeling
long-term: done for a long time
mental functioning: brain activity
miscarriage: too early delivery of a fetus
moderate: medium
molasses: brown sugar syrup
momentum: increased acceptance
nicotine: addictive chemical in tobacco
nonusers: those who don't use
noxious stimulus: unpleasant, offensive cause
numbness: no feeling
obesity: overweight, fat
on occasion: once in a while
opponents: those who disagree
paralysis: inability to move
paralyzing: causing to not move
peers: people of similar age, status
pleasant lift: good feeling
plug: large piece of tobacco
pollutant: something which makes air or water harmful
psychoactive: chemicals which affect mental states
puff: breath of smoke
quid: thick piece
quitters: people who stop something
rapidly: very fast, quickly
receding: pulling back
recommended: suggested as a good idea
relapse: starting a bad habit again

respiratory rate:	rate of breathing
roommate:	person who shares a living space
saliva:	moisture in the mouth
secretions:	leaking
sensitive:	easily affected
severe:	strong
smoker's breath:	bad breath caused by smoking
substantial:	large
sudden:	unexpected, quick
theoretically:	assumed
tobacco industry:	companies which make, sell tobacco
vessels:	blood veins
weaken:	make weak
weaned:	to give up a habit
wheezing:	difficult, noisy breathing
widespread:	spread over large area
withdrawal symptoms:	bad feelings from stopping something

CHAPTER 13
ILLICIT DRUGS: USE, MISUSE, AND ABUSE

Chapter Overview

Illicit drugs are illegal to possess, produce, and sell. Although the use of illicit drugs has seen a significant decline in recent years, usage is still quite high. Antidrug programs have been developed to deal with the problems of illegal drug use. The major drawback of most of these programs has been their failure to take a multidimensional approach.

In order to combat the increased use of illegal drugs and the overuse of certain prescription drugs, Congress passed the Controlled Substances Act of 1970. This law created categories for both prescription and illegal substances for which the federal government required strict regulation. Hundreds of illegal drugs exist. For general purposes, they can be divided into five categories: stimulants, marijuana and its derivatives, depressants, psychedelics and deliriants, and designer drugs. All are Schedule I or Schedule II drugs. These categories include drugs that are illegal to grow, manufacture, sell, or distribute in the United States. Cocaine is a crystallized white alkaloid powder derived from the leaves of the South American coca shrub. It is a very dangerous stimulant that can be taken in several ways: "snorted" through the nose, smoked, or injected intravenously. The amphetamines include a large and varied group of synthetic agents that stimulate the central nervous system. Newer-generation stimulants include methamphetamine, a powerfully addictive drug that strongly activates certain areas of the brain and affects the central nervous system as well. Marijuana is the most extensively used illicit drug by far. The long-term use of marijuana causes lung damage comparable to that caused by tobacco smoking. Marijuana has several medical purposes, such as to control the side effects of chemotherapy and to reduce the symptoms of glaucoma. Opiates cause drowsiness, relieve pain, and induce euphoria. Besides opium, they include morphine, codeine, heroin, and black tar heroin. Opiates are powerful central nervous system depressants, lowering heart rate, respiration, and blood pressure. Treatments for addiction to opiates have not been very successful. Methadone maintenance is controversial because of its addictive potential. Psychedelics are a group of drugs whose primary effect is to alter feelings, perceptions, and thoughts in the user. One psychedelic, lysergic acid diethylamide (LSD), is one of the most powerful drugs known to science. Deliriants produce confusion and disorientation at relatively low doses. Phencyclidine (PCP) is the best-known deliriant. Designer drugs are structural analogs of drugs already included under the Controlled Substances Act. These illegal drugs are manufactured by underground chemists to mimic the psychoactive effects of controlled drugs. Synthetic drugs available on the illegal drug market include analogs of PCP, analogs of fentanyl and meperidine, and analogs of amphetamine and methamphetamine. Inhalants are chemicals that produce hallucinogenic vapors, such as rubber cement, model glue, paint thinner, and lighter fluid. Anabolic steroids are artificial forms of the male hormone testosterone that produce muscle growth and strength. Several adverse effects occur in those who use steroids. They cause mood swings, acne, liver tumors, elevated cholesterol levels, hypertension, kidney disease, and immune system disturbances. There is also a danger of AIDS transmission through shared needles.

The financial burden of illegal drug use on the U.S. economy is staggering, with an estimated economic cost of almost $98 billion. Female addicts have special problems associated with seeking treatment. Estimates are that 9.2 percent of the total U.S. workforce consumes alcohol or drugs on any given workday. The use of mandatory drug urinalysis is controversial.

Researchers agree that a multimodal approach to drug education is best. Factual information works better than scare tactics. The best answer is education and self-discipline.

Learning Objectives

1. Discuss patterns of illicit drug use, including who uses illicit drugs and why they use them.

2. Describe the use and abuse of controlled substances, including cocaine, amphetamines, marijuana, opiates, psychedelics, deliriants, designer drugs, and inhalants.

3. Profile overall illegal drug use in the United States, including frequency, financial impact, arrests for drug offenses, and impact on the workplace.

Key Terms

Fill in a brief definition to help you remember these terms.

illicit drugs ______

cocaine ______

freebase ______

crack ______

ice ______

marijuana ______

tetrahydrocannabinol (THC) ______

hashish ______

narcotics ______

opium ______

morphine ______

codeine ______

heroin ______

black tar heroin ______

endorphins ______

methadone maintenance ______

psychedelics ______

reticular formation ______

synesthesia ____________________

hallucination ____________________

lysergic acid diethylamide (LSD) ____________________

mescaline ____________________

peyote ____________________

psilocybin ____________________

delirium ____________________

deliriant ____________________

phencyclidine (PCP) ____________________

designer drug ____________________

inhalants ____________________

amyl nitrite ____________________

nitrous oxide ____________________

anabolic steroids ____________________

ergogenic drug ____________________

Short Answers

1. What is the major drawback of most antidrug programs?

2. Which schedule of drugs has the highest potential for abuse?

3. List the criteria that determine under which schedule a substance is to be classified, according to the Controlled Substance Act.

4. Provide an example of a drug in each schedule.

5. Identify methods of cocaine use.

6. Name the most popular illicit drug.

7. What are the medical purposes of marijuana?

8. What group of drugs has as its primary pharmacological effect to alter the user's feelings, perceptions, and thoughts?

9. What are designer drugs?

10. What special problems might female addicts have when seeking treatment?

Critical Thinking Exercises

1. Theo entered a drug treatment program for cocajne use. In group therapy, he disclosed that he "shot up" cocaine. The group members shared their concerns for Theo's health. What are their concerns about his risk for infection and disease?

____

____

____

____

____

2. The use of mandatory drug analysis in the workplace is controversial. What is your opinion on this debate?

____

____

____

____

____

3. Roy is a heroin addict who is considering methadone maintenance treatment. Why is this treatment controversial?

____

____

____

____

____

4. Ellen is concerned that her roommate is using drugs. What are some indicators of drug abuse she should look for?

____

____

____

____

Critical Thinking Activity: The Question of Mandatory Drug Testing

Suppose that you have just been named chief executive officer of a ten million dollar corporation. The first decision you have to make is whether to require mandatory drug testing for your employees. You have a meeting with the head of the labor union representing the factory employees and the chairperson of the corporation's board of directors at which time you will announce your new policy. List the pros and cons of mandatory drug testing and summarize your conclusions as to whether mandatory drug testing will be instituted at your corporation.

Language Enrichment Glossary

In addition to the words in the Key Terms list at the end of the chapter, students listed the following words as difficult to understand. Use the chapter Key Terms list, this list, your dictionary, and teachers and friends to learn the meaning of words you do not understand.

accelerated: speeded up
adjunct: addition
adverse: negative
affinity: attraction to
alias: false name
alleviate: lessen
analgesics: pain-killers
analogs: similar substances
antisocial: unfriendly, hostile to others
atrophy: deteriorate, shrink to smaller size
attributable to: caused by
binds: attaches to

bizarre:	very strange
caught up:	involved in
coma:	unconscious condition
concerted:	strong
concoctions:	mixtures
contend:	say, believe
cravings:	desires
definitive:	absolute, definite
deliriants:	chemicals causing confusion, unconsciousness
dependence:	need to have something, addiction
derivative:	substance made from something else
derived:	developed from
dilapidated:	broken down, worn out
dilation:	opening up
directives:	rules, orders
emerge:	develop, become visible
entailed:	involved
erroneously:	incorrectly
exhibit:	show
hence:	therefore, because of this
hurdles:	barriers
illicit:	illegal
inconclusive:	no conclusion
instituted:	started
intravenous:	in the veins
introspective:	looking inward to the self
joint:	marijuana cigarette
justified:	done with good reason
mimic:	imitate
multimodal:	using many ways
negligible:	very small, unimportant
nostalgia:	good memories of the past
pales:	is minor
percolating:	dripping
potent:	strong
proponents:	those who agree with
relevant:	appropriate, related to
resolved:	settled
rush:	rapid good feeling
set and setting:	beliefs and surroundings
shoots up:	injects
snorts:	sniffs
spores:	tiny, single-cell seeds
surpassed:	greater than
syndrome:	group of symptoms of medical condition
synergistic:	effect cause by a combination of things
synthetic:	made by humans, not natural
viable:	realistic
volatile:	explodes easily

CHAPTER 14
NUTRITION: EATING FOR OPTIMUM HEALTH

Chapter Overview

Nutrition is the science that investigates the relationship between physiological functions and the essential elements of the foods we eat. Calories are eaten in the form of proteins, fats, and carbohydrates, three of the basic nutrients necessary for life. The Food Guide Pyramid, promoted by the U.S. Department of Agriculture, illustrates the importance of grains, cereals, vegetables, and fruits compared to meat, fish, poultry, dairy products, and other foods. It is a useful guide to daily food choices. Although eating the recommended number of servings from the food pyramid is important, you should be aware of nutrient density, or the caloric, fat, and energy differences between food categories within pyramid groups.

Water is necessary for human survival and maintenance of bodily functions. It is the most abundant substance in the human body, making up between 50 and 60 percent of our total body weight. Proteins are the essential constituents of nearly all body cells. Proteins are necessary for the development and repair of bone, muscle, skin, and blood, and are the key elements of antibodies, enzymes, and hormones. Carbohydrates are the major energy suppliers of the body. There are two major types of carbohydrates: simple sugars and complex carbohydrates. Fiber helps move foods through the digestive system and softens stools by absorbing large quantities of water. Fats are necessary for the maintenance of healthy skin and hair, insulation of body organs against shock, maintenance of body temperature, and the proper functioning of cells. However, fats must be consumed in moderation. Vitamins promote growth and help maintain life and health. Vitamins are either water soluble or fat soluble. Minerals aid physiological processes within the body. Without minerals, vitamins could not be absorbed. Although minerals are necessary for body function, there are limits to the amount we should consume. Americans tend to overuse or underuse certain minerals. Because men and women differ in body size, body composition, and overall metabolic rates, they have different nutritional needs throughout the life cycle.

Functional foods are based on the ancient belief that eating the right foods can not only prevent disease, but may actually cure diseases. Antioxidants have been heavily promoted in this decade. While antioxidants may, in fact, be beneficial, a conservative regimen will maximize their benefits. In 1998, the Food and Drug Administration (FDA) mandated folate fortification of all bread, cereal, rice and macaroni products sold in the United States. This practice is expected to decrease the number of infants born with spina bifida and other neural tube defects.

Between 5 and 15 percent of all Americans today claim to be vegetarians. If vegetarians combine the right types of food, they ensure proper nutrient intake. A food guide pyramid that conveys all the essentials of a vegetarian diet was devised in 1994 and was modeled after the Food Guide Pyramid. The vegetarian version clarifies what vegetarians need to eat to stay healthy.

College students often face a challenge when trying to eat healthy foods. But there are many tips for making healthy food choices. For instance, fast foods are not necessarily unhealthy. It is possible to eat healthy food by taking some simple steps, such as asking for nutritional analyses of items and ordering foods without the extras. To ensure a quality diet when funds are short, take steps such as using coupons, shopping at discount warehouse food chains, planning ahead to get the most for your dollar, and cooking large meals and freezing smaller portions for later use.

Food irradiation, food-borne illness, food additives, food allergies, and other food-safety concerns are becoming increasingly important to well-informed consumers. Learning potential risks and taking preventive measures are part of a good nutritional plan.

Learning Objectives

1. Examine the factors that influence your dietary decisions and discuss how you can change old eating habits, including appropriate use of the Food Guide Pyramid, eating nutrient-dense foods, and other factors.

2. Describe the major essential nutrients, indicating what purpose they serve in maintaining your overall health, as well as exploring many of the controversies that surround these substances.

3. Discuss the role of food as a form of medicine and the facts surrounding some of our newer foods and food supplements and their roles in health and well-being.

4. Distinguish among the various forms of vegetarianism, discussing possible health benefits and risks from these dietary alternatives.

5. Discuss issues surrounding gender and nutrition and explain the implications of some of these issues for your own dietary behaviors.

6. Discuss the unique problems that college students may have when trying to eat healthy foods and the actions that they can take to insure compliance with the food pyramid.

7. Explain some of the food safety concerns facing Americans as well as persons from other regions of the world.

Key Terms

Fill in a brief definition to help you remember these terms.

hunger ______________________________

appetite ______________________________

nutrition ______________________________

nutrients ______________________________

calorie ______________________________

digestive process ______________________________

saliva ______________________________

esophagus ______________________________

stomach ______________________________

small intestine ______________________________

dehydration ______________________________

proteins ______________________________

amino acids ______________________________

essential amino acids ______________________________

complete (high-quality) proteins ______________________________

incomplete proteins ______________________________

carbohydrates ______________________________

simple sugars ______________________________

complex carbohydrates ______________________________

monosaccharide ______________________________

disaccharide ______________________________

polysaccharide ______________________________

cellulose ______________________________

glycogen ______________________________

fats ______________________________

triglyceride ______________________________

cholesterol ______________________________

plaque ______________________________

high-density lipoproteins (HDLs) ______________________________

low-density lipoproteins (LDLs) ______________________________

saturated fats ______________________________

unsaturated fats ______________________________

vitamins ______________________________

hypervitaminosis ______________________________

minerals ______________________________

macrominerals ______________________________

trace minerals ______________________________

trans-fatty acids ______________________________

anemia ____

vegetarian ____

food irradiation ____

food allergies ____

food intolerance ____

organically grown ____

functional foods____

folate____

Recommended Daily Allowances (RDAs)______________________________

adequate intake ______________________________________

Short Answers

1. Define a calorie.

2. Explain how the digestive process works.

3. What are the two major types of carbohydrates?

4. What are the benefits of fiber?

5. Distinguish between high-density lipoproteins and low-density lipoproteins.

6. Distinguish between saturated and unsaturated fats.

7. Why do gender differences in nutritional needs exist?

8. What are organically grown foods and what problems do they have?

Critical Thinking Exercises

1. After reading this chapter, you no doubt have been able to decipher solid nutritional information from myths, untruths, and half-truths about a good nutritional plan. What are some of the myths you have held about nutrition? What information have you learned in this chapter that debunks these myths?

____

____

____

____

____

2. Suppose you are a nutritionist for a residence hall and have been asked to explain to the cafeteria staff how to ensure that students receive the essential nutrients. Explain to the staff how students can obtain the necessary water, proteins, carbohydrates, fiber, fats, vitamins, and minerals.

____

____

____

____

____

3. Suppose you are a nutritionist in a hospital. A patient who is ready to be discharged needs to reduce his fat intake. What guidelines will help him to reduce his fat intake?

4. John is a truck driver and eats a lot while on the road. He is concerned about how healthy his food choices are at fast food restaurants. What suggestions do you have that will ensure John's healthy eating?

5. A social worker is helping a single mother and her three children maintain nutritional eating, despite a lack of funds. What steps can this family take to ensure a quality diet?

Critical Thinking Activity: A Menu of Food Choices

The development of the Food Pyramid was designed to illustrate the importance of grains, cereals, vegetables, and fruits compared to meat, fish, poultry, dairy products, and other foods. It serves as a guide to daily food choices. In order to better understand the importance of good nutrition, develop your own menu of food choices for one week using the Food Pyramid as your guide.

MENU

****

Sunday

Breakfast

Bread, Cereal, Rice, and Pasta Group-
Vegetable Group-
Fruit Group-
Milk, Yogurt, and Cheese Group-
Meat, Poultry, Fish, Dry Beans, Eggs, and Nuts Group-
Fats, Oils, and Sweets-

Lunch

Bread, Cereal, Rice, and Pasta Group-
Vegetable Group-
Fruit Group-
Milk, Yogurt, and Cheese Group-
Meat, Poultry, Fish, Dry Beans, Eggs, and Nuts Group-
Fats, Oils, and Sweets-

Supper

Bread, Cereal, Rice, and Pasta Group-
Vegetable Group-
Fruit Group-
Milk, Yogurt, and Cheese Group-
Meat, Poultry, Fish, Dry Beans, Eggs, and Nuts Group-
Fats, Oils, and Sweets-

****

Monday

Breakfast

Bread, Cereal, Rice, and Pasta Group-
Vegetable Group-
Fruit Group-
Milk, Yogurt, and Cheese Group-
Meat, Poultry, Fish, Dry Beans, Eggs, and Nuts Group-
Fats, Oils, and Sweets-

Lunch

Bread, Cereal, Rice, and Pasta Group-
Vegetable Group-
Fruit Group-
Milk, Yogurt, and Cheese Group-
Meat, Poultry, Fish, Dry Beans, Eggs, and Nuts Group-
Fats, Oils, and Sweets-

Supper

Bread, Cereal, Rice, and Pasta Group-
Vegetable Group-
Fruit Group-
Milk, Yogurt, and Cheese Group-
Meat, Poultry, Fish, Dry Beans, Eggs, and Nuts Group-
Fats, Oils, and Sweets-

****

Tuesday

Breakfast

Bread, Cereal, Rice, and Pasta Group-
Vegetable Group-
Fruit Group-
Milk, Yogurt, and Cheese Group-
Meat, Poultry, Fish, Dry Beans, Eggs, and Nuts Group-
Fats, Oils, and Sweets-

Lunch

Bread, Cereal, Rice, and Pasta Group-
Vegetable Group-
Fruit Group-
Milk, Yogurt, and Cheese Group-
Meat, Poultry, Fish, Dry Beans, Eggs, and Nuts Group-
Fats, Oils, and Sweets-

Supper

Bread, Cereal, Rice, and Pasta Group-
Vegetable Group-
Fruit Group-
Milk, Yogurt, and Cheese Group-
Meat, Poultry, Fish, Dry Beans, Eggs, and Nuts Group-
Fats, Oils, and Sweets-

****

Wednesday

Breakfast

Bread, Cereal, Rice, and Pasta Group-
Vegetable Group-
Fruit Group-
Milk, Yogurt, and Cheese Group-
Meat, Poultry, Fish, Dry Beans, Eggs, and Nuts Group-
Fats, Oils, and Sweets-

Lunch

Bread, Cereal, Rice, and Pasta Group-
Vegetable Group-
Fruit Group-
Milk, Yogurt, and Cheese Group-
Meat, Poultry, Fish, Dry Beans, Eggs, and Nuts Group-
Fats, Oils, and Sweets-

Supper

Bread, Cereal, Rice, and Pasta Group-
Vegetable Group-
Fruit Group-
Milk, Yogurt, and Cheese Group-
Meat, Poultry, Fish, Dry Beans, Eggs, and Nuts Group-
Fats, Oils, and Sweets-

****

Thursday

Breakfast

Bread, Cereal, Rice, and Pasta Group-
Vegetable Group-
Fruit Group-
Milk, Yogurt, and Cheese Group-
Meat, Poultry, Fish, Dry Beans, Eggs, and Nuts Group-
Fats, Oils, and Sweets-

Lunch

Bread, Cereal, Rice, and Pasta Group-
Vegetable Group-
Fruit Group-
Milk, Yogurt, and Cheese Group-
Meat, Poultry, Fish, Dry Beans, Eggs, and Nuts Group-
Fats, Oils, and Sweets-

Supper

Bread, Cereal, Rice, and Pasta Group-
Vegetable Group-
Fruit Group-
Milk, Yogurt, and Cheese Group-
Meat, Poultry, Fish, Dry Beans, Eggs, and Nuts Group-
Fats, Oils, and Sweets-

****

Friday

Breakfast

Bread, Cereal, Rice, and Pasta Group-
Vegetable Group-
Fruit Group-
Milk, Yogurt, and Cheese Group-
Meat, Poultry, Fish, Dry Beans, Eggs, and Nuts Group-
Fats, Oils, and Sweets-

Lunch

Bread, Cereal, Rice, and Pasta Group-
Vegetable Group-
Fruit Group-
Milk, Yogurt, and Cheese Group-
Meat, Poultry, Fish, Dry Beans, Eggs, and Nuts Group-
Fats, Oils, and Sweets-

Supper

Bread, Cereal, Rice, and Pasta Group-
Vegetable Group-
Fruit Group-
Milk, Yogurt, and Cheese Group-
Meat, Poultry, Fish, Dry Beans, Eggs, and Nuts Group-
Fats, Oils, and Sweets-

****

Saturday

Breakfast

Bread, Cereal, Rice, and Pasta Group-
Vegetable Group-
Fruit Group-
Milk, Yogurt, and Cheese Group-
Meat, Poultry, Fish, Dry Beans, Eggs, and Nuts Group-
Fats, Oils, and Sweets-

Lunch

Bread, Cereal, Rice, and Pasta Group-
Vegetable Group-
Fruit Group-
Milk, Yogurt, and Cheese Group-
Meat, Poultry, Fish, Dry Beans, Eggs, and Nuts Group-
Fats, Oils, and Sweets-

Supper

Bread, Cereal, Rice, and Pasta Group-
Vegetable Group-
Fruit Group-
Milk, Yogurt, and Cheese Group-
Meat, Poultry, Fish, Dry Beans, Eggs, and Nuts Group-
Fats, Oils, and Sweets-

****

Questions for the Critical Thinker

After you have completed your menu, reflect on the following questions. Your thoughtful responses will enhance your learning of this critical thinking activity as well as your understanding of nutrition.

1. What did you learn about your nutritional choices from preparing a menu?

2. Was it easy or difficult to get all the recommended servings in each food group?

3. What changes do you need to make in your diet to ensure that you meet the pyramid requirements?

4. What modifications in food preparation can you make to use fats, oils, and sweets sparingly?

Language Enrichment Glossary

In addition to the words in the Key Terms list at the end of the chapter, students listed the following words as difficult to understand. Use the Key Terms list, this list, your dictionary, and teachers and friends to learn the meaning of words you do not understand.

adverse: negative
bombard: heavy attack
bulges: swellings
clarifies: makes clear
constipation: unable to make bowel movement
constraints: limits
convert: change
cravings: desires
crucial: very important, critical
dire: threatening, serious
discriminating: choosing carefully
duped: fooled, tricked
entice: tempt
essential: necessary
get it together: be organized, behave well
inception: beginning
junkie: someone addicted to something
landmark: important stage of development
maligned: criticized
mounting: increasing
optimum: maximum
pesticides: chemicals used to kill insects
pose: present
potent: strong
pouches: small pockets
preliminary: introductory
residual: remaining, left over
resounding: strong
skim milk: milk with most of the fat removed
skimp: economize, cut back on
soluble: easily dissolved in liquid
soy milk: drink made from soybean liquid
stem: come from

CHAPTER 15

MANAGING YOUR WEIGHT: FINDING A HEALTHY BALANCE

Chapter Overview

Knowing what weight is right for you depends on a number of variables, including body structure, height, the distribution of the weight that you carry, and the ratio of fat to lean tissue in your body. Obesity is defined as an accumulation of fat beyond what is considered normal for a person's age, sex, and body type. The difficulty with defining obesity is that there are no universally accepted standards for the ideal body weight or body composition. There are a variety of methods available for assessing your body content, including waist-to-hip ratios, hydrostatic weighing techniques, pinch and skinfold measures, girth and circumference measures, body mass index, soft-tissue roentgenogram, bioelectrical impedence analysis, and total body electrical conductivity.

There are many possible causes of obesity, including: heredity, hunger, appetite, and satiety mechanisms, excessive number of fat cells, setpoint theory, endocrine influence, psychosocial factors, eating cues, lack of awareness, metabolic changes, lifestyle, individuality, and the role of gender.

The two ways to lose weight are to decrease caloric intake and to increase exercise. Increasing your basal metabolic rate, your resting metabolic rate, or your exercise metabolic rate will help burn calories. Most health authorities recommend that, rather than going on a diet, a person should adopt nutritional dietary changes and a program of increased activity aimed at changing metabolic rates and increasing muscle strength. Improving the way you eat involves breaking old habits. First, determine what triggers your eating behavior. Usually, these dietary "triggers" center on problems in everyday living rather than real hunger pangs. Keeping a detailed diary of the triggers will help you understand what causes you to want food. Once you recognize the factors, removing the triggers or substituting other activities for them will help you develop more healthy eating patterns. Successful weight control includes setting realistic goals, such as trying to lose a healthy 1 to 2 pounds a week, seeking help from reputable sources in selecting a dietary plan, and avoiding fasting, starvation diets, and very low calorie diets. Some people are chronically underweight for metabolic, hereditary, or other reasons. Strategies for putting on needed pounds include reducing exercise, eating more high calorie foods, supplementing your diet with healthy high caloric drinks, and learning to relax.

Persons suffering from eating disorders have such an extreme fear of being fat that they engage in behaviors such as self-starvation, bingeing, vomiting, excessive exercise, and/or purging. Anorexia nervosa is characterized by self-starvation motivated by an intense fear of gaining weight along with a distorted body image to achieve weight loss. Bulimia nervosa is characterized by binge eating followed by inappropriate compensating measures taken to prevent weight gain. Binge eating refers to recurrent binge eating without excessive measures to lose the weight gained during binges. Treatment often focuses on reducing the threat to life and, once the patient is stabilized, long-term therapy, involving the family, friends, and other significant people in the individual's life. Therapy focuses on the psychological, social, environmental, and physiological factors that have led to the problem.

Learning Objectives

1. Describe those factors that place people at risk for problems with obesity. Indicate which factors are within your control and which are not.

2. Describe the options that are available for body content assessment. Indicate which are the most reliable and the possible shortcomings of each.

3. Discuss the roles of exercise, dieting, nutrition, lifestyle modification, fad diets and other strategies in weight control.

4. Indicate why so many diets fail and describe the most effective methods of weight management.

Key Terms
Fill in a brief definition to help you remember these terms.

obesity ____________________

hydrostatic weighing techniques ____________________

pinch test ____________________

skinfold caliper test ____________________

girth and circumference measures ____________________

body mass index (BMI) ____________________

soft-tissue roentgenogram ____________________

bioelectrical impedence analysis (BIA) ____________________

total body electrical conductivity unit (TOBEC) ____________________

adaptive thermogenesis ____________________

brown fat cells ____________________

hunger ____________________

appetite ____________________

satiety ____________________

hyperplasia ____________________

hypertrophy ____________________

setpoint theory ____________________

plateau ____________________

thyroid gland ____________________

basal metabolic rate (BMR) ____________________

yo-yo diet ____________________

resting metabolic rate (RMR) ____________________

exercise metabolic rate (EMR) ____________________

very low calorie diets (VLCDs) ____________________

ketosis ____

anorexia nervosa ____

bulimia nervosa ____

binge eating disorder (BED) ____

Short Answers

1. How has obesity been redefined?

2. What is the recommended range for body fat percentage in men and in women?

3. Distinguish between essential fat and storage fat.

4. Identify and explain one technique for assessing your body content.

5. Identify risk factors for obesity.

6. Distinguish between hunger and appetite.

7. What factors influence the basal metabolic rate?

8. List five tips for managing your weight.

9. What is the danger in very low calorie diets?

10. List the criteria for bulimia nervosa.

Critical Thinking Exercises

1. Kira is a 22-year-old college student. She goes to the health center for a weight assessment. She tells the technician that she is 5'6" and 135 pounds. What is Kira's body mass index? Is she in a desirable range?

2. At 140 pounds, Rhonda went on a diet to lose 25 pounds. When she dropped to 130 pounds, she still wanted to lose 15 more pounds to meet her goal. But she found that she had difficulty losing any additional weight. How does the setpoint theory explain Rhonda's difficulty with losing weight?

3. Forty-year-old Brenda decides that she needs to change her eating habits. What steps can she take to determine what triggers her eating? How can she remove the triggers or substitute other activities for them to help her develop more sensible eating patterns?

____

____

____

____

____

4. What triggers your "eat" response? What stops your "eat" response?

____

____

____

____

____

Critical Thinking Activity: How Healthy Are Your Eating Habits?

Assessing your eating attitudes and behaviors will help identify if you are in danger of developing anorexia nervosa or bulimia nervosa. The majority of persons suffering from an eating disorder are female. Answer the following questions carefully.

*Do I refuse to maintain my body weight over a minimal normal weight for my age and height?

*Am I afraid of gaining weight or becoming fat, even though I have been told that I am underweight?

*Do I often "feel fat"?

*Do I have amenorrhea?

*Do I engage in recurrent episodes of binge eating (eating a large amount of food in a discrete period of time)?

*Do I feel out of control over my eating behavior during the eating binges?

*Do I regularly engage in self-induced vomiting in order to prevent weight gain?

*Do I regularly use laxatives or diuretics in order to prevent weight gain?

*Do I regularly fast or am I on a strict diet in order to prevent weight gain?

*Do I engage in vigorous exercise in order to prevent weight gain?

*Do I have at least two binge eating episodes a week for the duration of at least three months?

*Am I consistently overconcerned about my body shape and weight?

If you answered yes to one or more of these questions, you may be at risk for developing an eating disorder. Consult with a counselor, an eating disorder clinic, a local hospital, or your college student health center for more information.

Language Enrichment Glossary

In addition to the words in the Key Terms list at the end of the chapter, students listed the following words as difficult to understand. Use the chapter Key Terms list, this list, your dictionary, and teachers and friends to learn the meaning of words you do not understand.

abound: overflow
appreciably: significantly
bingeing: uncontrolled eating
bolstered: encouraged
chronically: persistently, repeatedly
composed: made up of
comprehensive: complete, thorough
controversial: contradictory, debatable
corset: tight undergarment to shape breasts, waist and hips
credentials: qualifications
deplete: to consume
designated: specified
diminish: reduce
elect: choose
equated: associated
errant: abnormal
essence: basically
exemplify: represent
gluttony: excessive appetite
host: large number
mechanics: processes
mesmerized: fascinated by
morbidly: extremely unhealthful
organic: physical
phenomenon: occurrence, happening
plateau: level point
plausibility: believability
predispose: create a tendency toward
predominance: common occurrence
premises: guidelines
preoccupation: constant thoughts about
proponents: supporters
qualitative: regarding quality
quantitative: regarding quantity
quest: search
rational: realistic

reappraisal:	reassessment
reputable:	good reputation
sabotage:	undermine, disable
satiety:	fullness
sedentary:	inactive
slap in the face:	rejection, insult
sloth:	inactivity, laziness
sophisticated:	refined, complex

CHAPTER 16
PERSONAL FITNESS: IMPROVING YOUR HEALTH THROUGH EXERCISE

Chapter Overview

Regular physical activity improves more than 50 various metabolic, physiological, and psychological aspects of human life. Physiological rewards of exercise include improved cardiorespiratory fitness, improved bone mass, improved weight control, and improved health and life span. Psychological rewards of exercise include increased ability to cope with stress and improved self-esteem. Physical fitness is measured by cardiorespiratory endurance, flexibility, muscular strength, and muscular endurance.

The main category of physical activity known to enhance cardiorespiratory fitness is aerobic exercise. You will need to adjust the frequency, intensity, and duration of your aerobic activity program to accommodate your level of cardiorespiratory endurance. The Surgeon General's recommendation is for moderate amounts of *daily* physical activity. Monitoring exercise intensity is important. A target heart rate of 70 percent of maximum is known as the "conversational level of exercise" because you are able to talk with a partner while exercising. If you can sustain a conversational level of aerobic exercise for 20 to 30 minutes, you will improve your cardiorespiratory fitness. The Centers for Disease Control and Prevention (CDC) and the American College of Sports Medicine (ACSM) suggest that every adult engage in 20 to 60 minutes of continuous or intermittent (if intermittent, bouts of at least 10-minute duration) of moderate-intensity physical activity over the course of most days of the week.

Flexibility is a measure of the range of motion, or the amount of movement possible, at a particular joint. The three major types of stretching techniques are static, proprioceptive neuromuscular facilitation (PNF), and ballistic. Of these three, static stretches are most commonly used.

Muscular strength and endurance are maximized by following three key principles: the tension principle, the overload principle, and the specificity of training principle. Your skeletal muscles act in three different modes--isometric, concentric, and eccentric. There are four commonly used methods of applying resistance to develop strength and endurance: body weight, fixed, variable, and accommodating resistance.

The most frequent cause of injury associated with fitness activities is overtraining. There are two basic types of injuries caused by participation in fitness-related activities: overuse and traumatic. For personal fitness activities, appropriate exercise clothing and equipment are essential. Three of the most frequent injuries from repetitive overuse during exercise are plantar fascitis, shin splints, and runner's knee. First-aid treatment for virtually all personal fitness injuries involves rest, ice, compression, and elevation. Exercising in extreme temperatures heightens your risk for a heat-related injury. The three different heat stress illnesses are progressive in their level of severity: heat cramps, heat exhaustion, and heat stroke. When you exercise in cool to cold weather, especially in windy conditions, your body's rate of heat loss is frequently greater than its rate of heat production. Under these conditions, hypothermia may result. You can help prevent heat stress illnesses and hypothermia by following certain precautions.

Planning your fitness program involves setting your fitness goals and designing your fitness program so that it is best suited to your needs.

Learning Objectives

1. Describe the benefits of regular physical activity, including improved cardiorespiratory fitness, muscular fitness, bone mass, weight control, stress management, mental health, and lifespan.

2. Describe the components of an aerobic exercise program and how to determine proper exercise frequency, intensity, and duration.

3. Describe the different stretching exercises designed to improve flexibility.

4. Compare the various types of resistance exercise programs, including the methods of providing external resistance and intended physiological benefits.

5. Describe common fitness injuries, suggest ways to prevent injuries, and list the treatment process.

6. Summarize the key components of a personal fitness program.

Key Terms

Fill in a brief definition to help you remember these terms.

systolic blood pressure ______________________________

diastolic blood pressure ______________________________

osteoporosis ______________________________

physical fitness ______________________________

exercise training ______________________________

cardiorespiratory fitness ______________________________

aerobic exercise ______________________________

aerobic capacity ______________________________

graded exercise test ______________________________

target heart rate ______________________________

flexibility ______________________________

tai chi ______________________________

yoga ______________________________

isometric muscle action ______________________________

concentric muscle action ______________________________

eccentric muscle action ______________________________

static stretching ______________________________

ballistic stretching ______________________________

muscular strength ______________________________

one repetition maximum (1RM) ____________________

muscular endurance ____________________

resistance exercise program ____________________

hypertrophy ____________________

overuse injuries ____________________

traumatic injuries ____________________

RICE ____________________

heat cramps ____________________

heat exhaustion ____________________

heat stroke ____________________

hypothermia ____________________

cross training ____________________

Short Answers

1. List six physiological benefits of regular exercise.

2. Name the four components of physical fitness.

3. Provide three examples of aerobic activity.

4. What are the three components of aerobic fitness programs?

5. What are three major types of stretching techniques? Which of these techniques is most commonly used?

6. What three principles do you need to follow in order to improve your muscular strength?

7. Identify and define the three types of muscle activity.

8. What are two basic types of injuries that can result from participation in fitness-related activities?

9. What are three common overuse injuries?

Critical Thinking Exercises

1. Alayna has just begun a regular exercise program at a fitness center. What psychological benefits can she expect to gain by engaging in regular physical activity?

____

____

____

____

____

:. David is 35 years old. He is monitoring his exercise intensity during aerobic exercise. David wants to exercise .t 70 percent of his maximum heart rate. What is his target heart rate? How can David determine how close he is to his value during his workout?

. What activity could you engage in to apply body weight resistance? fixed resistance? variable resistance? ccommodating resistance?

Andre sprained his ankle during a one-on-one basketball game. Explain how to apply the first-aid treatment iown as RICE to Andre's ankle.

Using the Activity Pyramid as a guide (refer to Figure 11.2), create your own pyramid. List your daily activities, tivities you engage in 3-5 times a week, activities you engage in 2-3 times a week, and activities you need to cut wn on. You may also list new activities you would like to start. Each week, try to increase your physical activity ing your personal guide.

Critical Thinking Activity: Planning My Personal Fitness Program

Plan your own fitness program. Use the following worksheet to help you design a fitness program that meets your individual needs.

PLANNING MY PERSONAL FITNESS PROGRAM

What is my primary reason for exercising?

____

What are my fitness goals? (short-term and long-term goals)

____

____

____

What type of fitness program is best suited to my needs? (amount of exercise, type of exercise)

____

____

____

Do I need to consult my physician before I begin my fitness program?

____

What exercise clothing and equipment do I need?

____

____

Good fitness programs are designed to improve or maintain fitness in all four major components of physical fitness. What will I include in my comprehensive program?

____

____

The following schedule is what I choose for an exercise program:

<u>Sunday</u>
Type of exercise

Frequency of exercise

Duration of exercise

Location of exercise

<u>Monday</u>
Type of exercise

Frequency of exercise

Duration of exercise

Location of exercise

<u>Tuesday</u>
Type of exercise

Frequency of exercise

Duration of exercise

Location of exercise

<u>Wednesday</u>
Type of exercise

Frequency of exercise

Duration of exercise

Location of exercise

<u>Thursday</u>
Type of exercise

Frequency of exercise

Duration of exercise

Location of exercise

Friday
Type of exercise

Frequency of exercise

Duration of exercise

Location of exercise

Saturday
Type of exercise

Frequency of exercise

Duration of exercise

Location of exercise

Language Enrichment Glossary

In addition to the words in the Key Terms list at the end of the chapter, students listed the following words as difficult to understand. Use the chapter Key Terms list, this list, your dictionary, and teachers and friends to learn the meaning of words you do not understand.

absorbency: ability to absorb
accelerating: speeding up
acclimatization: becoming used to
accommodate: fit
adequate: enough
afflicted: to suffer from
alters: changes
apathy: inactivity, disinterest
arch: raised middle of foot bottom
attain: to reach
bouts: periods
briskly: actively
buoyancy: ability to hold up
cadence: pattern
celebrity: famous person, star
colon: intestine
compartments: parts
component: part
concept: idea
coronary: heart
curl: lifting weights
current: up-to-date
customizes: adjusts to fit
debilitating: weakening

desire: strong want
despair: to give up
detrimental: harmful
dormant: inactive
duration: period of time
efficiency: smooth, not wasteful
embark: begin
exertion: effort
expenditure: payment
external: outside
extremities: arms and legs
facets: sides
facial: on the face
fatiguing: tiring
flexed: bent
flexion: moving or flexing muscles
flotation device: object to help a person float in water
goggles: protective glasses
goosebumps: skin bumps caused by feeling cold or scared
hard task: difficult job
hinder: get in the way of
immersion: covered by water
initiating: starting
integral: central
intensity: power
interdependent: affect each other
leveled off: stopped increasing
light: not much, not heavy
load: burden, amount of work
midsole: middle of shoe sole
moderate: medium
modes: ways
modifications: changes
monotonous: repetitive, boring
novice: newcomer
obesity: overweight
osteoporosis: bone deterioration
overdoing: doing too much
overload: too large a burden
padded grips: padding on handles
paradoxically: contradictory
portability: easy to carry
postures: way of holding the body
predictor: estimate
prudent: careful
range of motion: ability to move
receptors: receivers
resiliency: adaptability, flexibility
retention: holding
reusable: can be used repeatedly

sampling:	trying
segment:	part
sequential:	step by step
sporadically:	from time to time
squats:	bending at the knees
stemming:	coming from
systematic:	organized
tension:	force, pulling
terrain:	land
treadmill:	stationary walking device for exercise
vigorous:	strong, active
vows:	promises

CHAPTER 17
CARDIOVASCULAR DISEASE: HELPING THE BEAT GO ON

Chapter Overview

Cardiovascular diseases (CVDs) are the leading cause of death in the United States today, accounting for 42 percent of all deaths. You can reduce your risk for CVD by taking steps to change certain behaviors. It is important to know how the cardiovascular system functions. The cardiovascular system is the network of elastic tubes through which blood flows as it carries oxygen and nutrients to all parts of the body. The four chambers of the heart work together to ensure that blood is constantly recirculated to body parts. For the heart to function properly, the four chambers must beat in an organized manner. The average adult heart at rest beats 70 to 80 times per minute. When overly stressed, a heart may beat over 200 times per minute, especially in an individual who is overweight or out of shape. A healthy heart functions more efficiently and is less likely to suffer damage from overwork than is an unhealthy one.

The most common forms of heart disease include atherosclerosis, heart attack, chest pain, irregular heartbeat, congestive heart failure, congenital and rheumatic heart disease, and stroke. Prevention and treatment of these diseases range from changes in diet and lifestyle to use of medications and surgery.

Risk factors for cardiovascular disease are divided into two types: those that can be controlled and those that cannot. Things that you can do to reduce your risk for CVD include: stop smoking, cut down on fats and cholesterol, cut back on overall triglycerides, monitor your cholesterol levels, control your blood pressure, exercise, lose weight, control diabetes risks, and manage stress. Risks you cannot control include heredity, age, gender, and race.

While men do have more heart attacks and have them earlier in life, women have a low chance of surviving a heart attack. Premenopausal women are unlikely candidates for heart attacks, except for those who suffer from diabetes, high blood pressure, kidney disease, or who have a genetic predisposition to high cholesterol levels. Family history and smoking can also increase the risk for premenopausal women. Once her estrogen production drops with menopause, a woman's chances of developing CVD rise rapidly. Symptoms of heart disease in postmenopausal women often are manifested differently than in men. Research suggests three main reasons for the widespread neglect of the signs of heart disease in women: physicians may be gender-biased, physicians tend to view male heart disease as a more severe problem, and women decline major procedures more often than do men.

Several methods are used to diagnose heart disease, including electrocardiogram, angiography, and positron emission tomography scans. New methods developed for treating heart blockages include radionuclide imaging, magnetic resonance imaging, and digital cardiac angiography. During the 1980s, coronary bypass surgery seemed to be the ultimate method for treating patients who had coronary blockages or who had suffered heart attacks. Recently, experts have begun to question the effectiveness of bypass operations, particularly for elderly people. A procedure called angioplasty is associated with fewer risks and is believed by many experts to be more effective than bypass surgery in selected cardiovascular cases. Research has indicated that the use of low-dose aspirin is beneficial to heart patients. However, gastrointestinal intolerance is a major problem associated with aspirin use, as well as a tendency for some people to have difficulty with blood clotting, and these factors may outweigh its benefits for some people. If a heart attack occurs, and a victim gets to an emergency room fast enough, a form of reperfusion therapy called thrombolysis can sometimes be performed.

Learning Objectives

1. Discuss the incidence, prevalence and outcomes of CVD in America, including the impact of CVD on society.

2. Describe the anatomy and physiology of the heart and circulatory system and the importance of healthy heart functioning.

3. Review the various types of heart disease, factors that contribute to their development, current diagnostic and treatment options, as well as the importance of fundamental lifestyle modifications aimed at prevention.

4. Discuss the controllable risk factors for cardiovascular disease, including smoking, cholesterol and triglycerides, certain infectious organisms, diet and obesity, exercise, hypertension, diabetes mellitus, and stress. Examine your own risk profile and determine those you can and cannot control.

5. Discuss the issues surrounding CVD risk and disease burden from the perspective of women and persons from diverse backgrounds.

6. Discuss some of the newer methods of diagnosing and treating CVD, and the importance of being a wise health care consumer when facing various options for CVD risk reduction.

Key Terms

Fill in a brief definition to help you remember these terms.

cardiovascular diseases (CVDs) ____________________

cardiovascular system ____________________

atria ____________________

ventricles ____________________

arteries ____________________

arterioles ____________________

capillaries ____________________

veins ____________________

sinoatrial node (SA node) ____________________

atherosclerosis ____________________

arteriosclerosis ____________________

plaque ____________________

myocardial infarction (MI) ____________________

heart attack ____________________

coronary thrombosis ____________________

collateral circulation ____________________

ischemia ______________________________

angina pectoris ______________________________

beta blockers ______________________________

arrhythmia ______________________________

fibrillation ______________________________

congenital heart disease ______________________________

rheumatic heart disease ______________________________

stroke ______________________________

thrombus ______________________________

embolus ______________________________

aneurysm ______________________________

transient ischemic attacks (TIAs) ______________________________

low-density lipoproteins (LDLs) ______________________________

high-density lipoproteins (HDLs) ______________________________

triglycerides ______________________________

hypertension ______________________________

essential hypertension ______________________________

secondary hypertension ______________________________

systolic pressure ______________________________

diastolic pressure ______________________________

hormone replacement therapies (HRTs) ______________________________

electrocardiogram (ECG) ______________________________

angiography ______________________________

positron emission tomography (PET scan) ______________________________

coronary bypass surgery ______________________________

angioplasty ____

thrombolysis ____

Short Answers

1. What behaviors can reduce an individual's risk for CVD?

2. Explain how the heart ensures that blood is constantly recirculating to body parts.

3. Name common types of cardiovascular disease.

4. Distinguish between tachycardia and bradycardia.

5. When blood supply to the brain is cut off, what disease occurs?

6. Identify risk factors for CVD that cannot be prevented or controlled.

7. Describe how the symptoms of heart disease are manifested differently in men and women.

8. List reasons for neglect of heart disease symptoms in women.

9. Identify and describe one technique for diagnosing heart disease.

10. What is a major problem associated with aspirin use to prevent heart disease?

Critical Thinking Exercises

1. Bob had a heart attack five years ago and his family has a history of heart disease. Bob's new wife wants to know how to be prepared in the event that Bob has another heart attack. List the warning signals of a heart attack and explain what she should do in the event of another heart attack.

____

____

____

____

____

2. Summarize ways to reduce risks for heart attack. Identify those that may apply to you.

____

____

____

____

____

3. Noreen just experienced menopause. Her doctor explained that once her estrogen production drops with menopause, her chances of developing CVD rise rapidly. Explain the role of estrogen as a risk factor for heart disease.

4. Jack suffered a coronary blockage. His doctor met with him to discuss his treatment. The doctor discussed two procedures: angioplasty and bypass surgery. What suggestions can you offer to Jack to ensure that he feels comfortable with his choice?

Critical Thinking Activity: Taking Responsibility for Your Health Risks

The causes of cardiovascular disease include lack of exercise, stress, high sodium intake, and high-fat diets. The incidence of CVD in this country could be cut substantially if people simply took better care of themselves. Noting this, answer the following questions:

1. Should public health care funds be reduced for people who have somehow contributed to their own medical condition? Why or why not?

2. Are there any such provisions in place now?

3. In what ways are individuals encouraged to take better care of themselves? Is there any financial incentive to take better care of yourself?

4. Do you think people are becoming more aware of the need for wellness programs? Why or why not?

Language Enrichment Glossary

In addition to the words in the Key Terms list at the end of the chapter, students listed the following words as difficult to understand. Use the Key Terms list, this list, your dictionary, and teachers and friends to learn the meaning of words you do not understand.

abnormalities: unexpected outcomes
aggressive: done with intensity, commitment
causal link: connection between cause and effect
chronic: periodic, long-lasting
comply with: agree to
compounded: increased
conflicting data: differing information
diagnostic: having to do with deciding the cause

diuretics:	substances that increase urination
emits:	to put out
enhance:	increase
gender-biased:	influenced by beliefs about one gender
governed:	regulated, supervised
insure:	guarantee
internalize:	keep inside
intolerance:	negative reaction, inability to tolerate
invasive:	intruding
longitudinal study:	study comparing information at different times
manifestation:	evidence, symptom
optimism:	cheerfulness, positive outlook
overwhelmed:	surprised, overcome
pacemaker:	mechanism that regulates heartbeats
pose:	present, cause
quivering:	shaking, trembling
readily:	easily
relative:	comparable
sedentary:	inactive
shove...in your face:	place something abruptly in front of you
site:	location
sporadic:	periodic, irregular
taxed:	overworked, strained
therapeutic:	treatment of an illness
unique challenge:	specific difficulty
warranted:	justified, called for

CHAPTER 18
CANCER: REDUCING YOUR RISKS

Chapter Overview

Cancer is the name given to a large group of diseases characterized by the uncontrolled growth and spread of abnormal cells. These cells may create tumors. Cancerous tumors are called malignant, while noncancerous tumors, the majority of tumors, are benign. A biopsy determines whether a given tumor or mass is benign or malignant.

Cancer is caused by both external and internal factors. Scientists have proposed several theories for the cellular changes that produce cancer, including spontaneous error, environmental carcinogens, and oncogenes. Some of the most widely suspected causes of cancer include lifestyle factors, biological factors, occupational/environmental factors, social and psychological factors, food chemicals, viral factors, and medical factors.

There are four broad classifications of cancer, depending upon the type of tissue from which the cancer arises. Carcinomas are in the epithelial tissues: sarcomas occur in the mesodermal, or middle, layers of tissue; lymphomas develop in the lymphatic system; and leukemia is cancer of the blood-forming parts of the body, particularly the bone marrow and spleen. Common cancers include those of the lung, breast, colon and rectum, prostate, skin, testicular, ovarian, endometrium, pancreas, and leukemia.

The sooner a person is diagnosed as having cancer, the better the prospect for survival. Various high-tech diagnostic techniques exist to detect cancer. These medical techniques, along with regular self-examinations and checkups, play an important role in the early detection and secondary prevention of cancer. Although cancer treatments have changed significantly over the last 20 years, surgery, in which the tumor and surrounding tissue are removed, is still common. Today's surgeons tend to remove less surrounding tissue than they did previously, and to combine surgery with either radiotherapy or chemotherapy to kill cancerous cells. Today, new treatments are focusing on cancer as a genetic disease. Treatments focus on stopping the cycle of these mutant cells, targeting toxins through monoclonal antibodies, and rousing the immune system to be more effective. Other advances in the treatment of cancer include the use of tamoxifen, immunotherapy, gene therapy, angiogenesis inhibitors, rational drug design, TIMP-2, and neoadjuvant chemotherapy.

Learning Objectives

1. Define cancer and discuss how cancer develops.
2. Discuss the probable causes of cancer, including biological causes, occupational and environmental causes, lifestyle, psychological causes, chemicals in foods, viral causes, medical causes, and combined causes.
3. Identify and describe several different types of cancer, each of which poses different risks to people at different ages and stages of life.
4. Facing cancer poses many challenges. Discuss how understanding and acting appropriately in response to self-exams, medical exams, and symptoms related to different types of cancers is an important element of successful cancer survival.
5. Discuss cancer detection and treatment, including radiation therapy, chemotherapy, immunotherapy and other common methods of detection and treatment in use today.

Key Terms
Fill in a brief definition to help you remember these terms.

cancer ______________________________

neoplasm ______________________________

tumor ______________________________

malignant ______________________________

benign ______________________________

biopsy ______________________________

metastasis ______________________________

mutant cells ______________________________

carcinogens ______________________________

oncogenes ______________________________

protooncogenes ______________________________

oncologists ______________________________

malignant melanoma ______________________________

PAP test ______________________________

magnetic resonance imaging (MRI) ______________________________

computerized axial tomography (CAT scan) ______________________________

prostate-specific antigen (PSA) ______________________________

radiotherapy ______________________________

chemotherapy ______________________________

immunotherapy ______________________________

Short Answers

1. How do benign and malignant tumors differ?

2. Explain the theory that suggests cancer is caused by oncogenes.

3. Name the four classifications of cancer.

4. What are warning signals of breast cancer? What are the risk factors for breast cancer?

5. What are symptoms of prostate cancer?

6. What are symptoms of skin cancer?

7. What are symptoms of ovarian cancer? What is the main risk factor for ovarian cancer?

8. What are early warning signs of endometrium (uterine) cancer?

9. How does radiation work in treating cancer?

10. Identify and describe one new procedure in cancer treatment.

Critical Thinking Exercises

1. Ever since Julien turned 30 and started a family, he has become concerned about his health. Since he has a family history of cancer, he is concerned about a diet that reduces his risk for cancer. According to the guidelines of the American Cancer Society, what steps can Julien take to reduce his risk?

2. Sandy believes that cancer detection is her responsibility. She should be aware of what seven warning signals for cancer?

3. Fifty-two-year-old Stan and 50-year-old Susan believe in taking responsibility for their health. They want to make sure that appropriate diagnostic tests for cancer are done. What tests should each have and how often should these tests be done?

Critical Thinking Activity: Reviewing Personal Risk Factors for Cancer

Describe six aspects of your life that tend to increase your risk for developing cancer, such as smoking. Identify why you engage in these high-risk behaviors, indicate whether you plan to change these behaviors, and list any measures you plan to take which could lower these risks.

Language Enrichment Glossary

In addition to the words in the Key Terms list at the end of the chapter, students listed the following words as difficult to understand. Use the chapter Key Terms list, this list, your dictionary, and teachers and friends to learn the meaning of words you do not understand.

acute:	severe
agent:	cause
at risk:	likely to get
avid:	eager, enthusiastic
benign:	not harmful
biopsy:	examination of a small piece of tissue
blood-streaked:	marked with blood
circumvent:	get around
conversely:	considering the opposite
counterparts:	similar people
cumulative:	total
curtailed:	limited, ended
demographically similar:	similar characteristics
fashion:	way
given:	specific
grad:	graduate
hazards:	dangers
heeding:	listening to

hemorrhaging: bleeding which doesn't stop
imaging: procedures for looking at something
incidence: occurrence
likelihood: probability
lobbied: pushed for
mammogram: breast x-ray
manifest: show up, develop
mechanisms: processes
monitoring: watching, checking
mortality rates: death rates
opportunistic: taking advantage of a situation
options: choices
oral cavity: mouth and upper throat
orthodox: traditional
particular: specific
prognosis: expectations of future health
programmed: set
prolonged: extended over a long time
prone: a tendency toward
proposes: suggests
readily: easily
regimen: treatment
routinely: usually
sites: locations
skeptical: not believing
socioeconomic: social and economic standing
sputum: mucus coughed up from the lungs
susceptibility: tendency to develop problem
suspect: suspicious
tampering: adjusting, changing
variability: variation
virulent: disease which spreads rapidly

CHAPTER 19
INFECTIOUS DISEASES AND SEXUALLY TRANSMITTED INFECTIONS: REDUCING RISKS AND INCREASING RESPONSIBILITIES

Chapter Overview

Most diseases are multifactorial. For a disease to occur, the host must be susceptible, an agent capable of transmitting a disease must be present, and the environment must be hospitable to the pathogen. Other risk factors also apparently increase or decrease levels of susceptibility. Some of the most common uncontrollable risk factors are heredity, aging, and environmental conditions. Controllable risk factors include too much stress, inadequate nutrition, a low physical fitness level, lack of sleep, misuse or abuse of legal and illegal substances, personal hygiene, and high-risk behaviors.

There are numerous ways that pathogens enter the body: direct contact, such as during sexual relations; indirect contact, such as by touching an object the infected person has had contact with; autoinoculation; airborne contact; food-borne infection; animal-borne pathogens; and water-borne diseases. The most common pathogens are bacteria, viruses, fungi, protozoa, and parasitic worms.

Body defenses include physical and chemical defenses, the immune system, fever, pain, vaccines, and active and passive immunity.

Today's antiobiotics appear to be increasingly ineffective, with penicillin-resistant strains of diseases on the rise as microbes are able to outlast even the best antibiotics available. The following lethal threats include: mad cow disease, dengue and dengue hemorrhagic fever, ebola, cryptosporidium, escherichia coli, cholera, hantavirus, and flesh-eating strep.

Today, there are over 20 different types of sexually transmitted infections (STIs). There are multiple reasons for these high rates. A stigma associated with these diseases often keeps infected people from seeking treatment, and these people usually continue to be sexually active, thereby infecting unsuspecting partners. People who are uncomfortable discussing sexual issues may also be less likely to use and/or ask their partners to use condoms as a means of protecting against STIs and/or pregnancy. Also, the casual attitude about sex that prevails today lends itself to not considering the consequences. In addition, many STIs are asymptomatic in some people and the infected person may unknowingly spread the disease to an unsuspecting partner. STIs are generally spread through some form of intimate sexual contact. Sexual intercourse, oral-genital contact, hand-genital contact, and anal intercourse are the most common modes of transmission. Chlamydia is one of the most commonly reported infections in the United States. Unfortunately, many chlamydia victims display no symptoms and therefore do not seek help until the disease has done secondary damage, which is serious in both sexes. Chlamydia can be controlled through responsible sexual behavior and familiarity with the early symptoms of the disease. If detected early enough, chlamydia is easily treatable with antibiotics. Pelvic inflammatory disease (PID) refers to a number of infections of the uterus, fallopian tubes, and ovaries. PID is often the result of an untreated sexually transmitted disease, but nonsexual causes of PID are also common, such as excessive vaginal douching or cigarette smoking. Gonorrhea primarily infects the linings of the urethra, genital tract, pharynx, and rectum. It may be spread to the eyes or other body regions via the hands or body fluids. The incidence of syphilis has been increasing in recent years in the United States. Left untreated, this disease progresses from the primary stage to the secondary, latent, and late stages, with devastating consequences. Treatment for syphilis is with antibiotics. The major obstacle to treatment is misdiagnosis of this "imitator" disease. Pubic lice are small parasites that are usually transmitted during sexual contact. Venereal warts are caused by human papilloma viruses (HPVs). A person becomes infected when an HPV penetrates the skin and mucous membranes of the genitals or anus through sexual contact. Candidiasis is a yeastlike fungus caused by the candida albicans organism that normally inhabits the vaginal tract in most women. Only under certain conditions will these organisms multiply to abnormal quantities and begin to cause problems. Trichomoniasis is caused by a protozoan. Although usually transmitted by sexual contact, the "trich" organism may be easily spread by toilet seats, wet towels, or other items that have discharged fluids on them. Some forms of general urinary tract infections are sexually transmitted. Herpes is a general term for a family of diseases characterized by sores or eruptions on the skin. Herpes simplex virus type 1 causes cold sores and fever blisters. Genital herpes is caused by herpes simplex virus type 2.

Although deaths due to Acquired Immune Deficiency Syndrome (AIDS) have decreased in the United States in the last few years, HIV/AIDS continues to be a significant global health threat. AIDS is caused by the human immunodeficiency virus (HIV). HIV is not an infection that affects certain groups because of inherent group characteristics, but rather, an equal-opportunity pathogen that can attack anyone who engages in certain high-risk behaviors. The HIV virus typically enters one person's body when another person's infected body fluids gain entry through a breach in body defenses. Mucous membranes of the genital organs and the anus provide the easiest route of entry. High-risk activities that are known to spread the virus include exchange of body fluids, receiving a blood transfusion prior to 1985, injecting drugs, and mother-to-infant transmission (perinatal). A person may go for months or years after infection by HIV before any significant symptoms appear. The incubation time varies greatly from person to person. Children have shorter incubation periods than do adults. The ELISA and Western blot tests detect antibodies of the disease, indicating the presence of the HIV in the person's system. New high-powered, anti-HIV drugs have slowed the progression from HIV to AIDS and have prolonged life expectancies in many AIDS patients. Of those that have gained approval, zidovudine (AZT) has been the mainstay of treatment. Protease inhibitors are a promising new class of antiretroviral therapies for the treatment of HIV infection. The only effective prevention strategies known all closely relate to the means by which people contract AIDS. You can reduce your risks by the choices you make in sexual behaviors and the responsibilities you take for your health and for that of your loved ones.

Learning Objectives

1. Discuss the risk factors for infectious diseases, including those you can control and those you cannot.

2. Describe the most common pathogens infecting humans today and summarize the major characteristics of the pathogen as well as the typical diseases caused by each pathogen.

3. Describe your immune system and how it works to protect you as well as those factors that may make your immune system work less effectively in protecting you from invading organisms.

4. Explain the major emerging and resurgent diseases affecting humans today; discuss why they are increasing in numbers and what actions we are taking to reduce risks.

5. Discuss the various sexually transmitted infections, their means of transmission, and actions that can be taken to prevent their spread.

6. Discuss Human Immunodeficiency Virus (HIV), and Acquired Immune Deficiency Syndrome, trends in infection, treatment, and the impact on special populations such as women and members of the international community.

Key Terms

Fill in a brief definition to help you remember these terms.

pathogen ______________________________

epidemic ______________________________

pandemics______________________________

virulent ______________________________

multifactorial disease ______________________________

sickle cell anemia ______________________________

immunological competence ______________________________

botulism______________________________

autoinoculation______________________________

interspecies transmission______________________________

bacteria______________________________

toxins______________________________

staphylococci ______________________________

epidermis ______________________________

toxic shock syndrome ______________________________

streptococci ______________________________

pneumonia ______________________________

tuberculosis (TB) ______________________________

periodontal diseases ______________________________

rickettsia ______________________________

viruses ______________________________

incubation period ______________________________

slow-acting viruses ______________________________

interferon ______________________________

endemic ______________________________

influenza ______________________________

hepatitis ______________________________

measles ______________________________

German measles (rubella) ______________________________

rabies ______________________________

asymptomatic ______________________________

fungi ______________________________

protozoa ______________________________

parasitic worms ______________________________

puons ______________________________

enzymes ______________________________

antigen ______________________________

antibodies ______________________________

referred pain ______________________________

vaccination ______________________________

acquired immunity ______________________________

natural immunity ______________________________

passive immunity ______________________________

sexually transmitted infections (STIs) ______________________________

chlamydia ______________________________

conjunctivitis ______________________________

pelvic inflammatory disease (PID) ______________________________

human papilloma virus (HPV) ______________________________

gonorrhea ______________________________

syphilis ______________________________

chancre ______________________________

pubic lice ______________________________

venereal warts ______________________________

candidiasis ______________________________

vaginitis ______________________________

trichomoniasis ______________________________

genital herpes ______________________________

acquired immune deficiency syndrome (AIDS) ______________________________

human immunodeficiency virus (HIV) ______________________________

ELISA ______________________________

western blot ______________________________

Short Answers

1. List three routes of invasion for pathogens and provide an example of each.

2. What steps can a woman take to reduce the likelihood of contracting toxic shock syndrome?

3. What are two examples of streptococcal infections?

4. What is one of the greatest dangers associated with mumps?

5. German measles, or rubella, is not a serious health threat and usually runs its course in 3 to 4 days. What are major exceptions to this statement?

6. Explain how the immune system works to defend against any invading organisms.

7. What is an example of an autoimmune disease?

8. Distinguish between acquired and natural immunity.

9. List reasons for the high rates of sexually transmitted infections (STIs).

10. What are the risk factors for pelvic inflammatory disease?

11. Describe the symptoms of syphilis in its various stages.

12. Identify high-risk behaviors for contracting AIDS.

Critical Thinking Exercises

1. List five controllable risk factors for infectious diseases. Which of these factors put you at risk? What do you need to change to lessen your risk for disease?

____

____

____

____

____

2. Janet is taking her newborn to the pediatrician. She is concerned about her baby receiving any vaccines because she doesn't understand how they work. How do vaccinations work? What vaccines are recommended in childhood?

3. Sarah is beginning to feel ill, but is not sure if she has a cold or the flu. Compare cold and flu symptoms.

4. Sasha has genital herpes. What can she do to prevent herpes in her sexual partner?

5. Ted has become concerned about contracting HIV disease. What can he do to reduce his risk for contracting the disease?

Critical Thinking Activity: Campaigning Against Risky Behaviors

AIDS is not a disease of certain groups. Rather, it is a disease of certain high-risk behaviors. The estimated number of cases worldwide reveal a disturbing lack of progress in HIV prevention. What campaign effort could be mounted to effectively convey this message to the general public? Outline your ideas below.

Language Enrichment Glossary

In addition to the words in the Key Terms list at the end of the chapter, students listed the following words as difficult to understand. Use the chapter Key Terms list, this list, your dictionary, and teachers and friends to learn the meaning of words you do not understand.

abstinence: avoidance
afflicted: infected
apathy: indifference
asymptomatic: without symptoms
autoinoculate: infect yourself
average: normal, ordinary
breach: cross
celibate: no sexual relations
cesarean delivery: surgical delivery
confidential: name kept secret
congenital: inherited
conquered: defeated
dealt: given
dirty blow: unfair behavior

excision:	cut out
frenzied:	violent agitation
grave:	serious
incubation:	development time
inherent:	inherited, built in
inheritance:	inherited from ancestors
inhospitable:	not welcoming
itchy:	tickles, needs scratching
jaundice:	liver disease
lesions:	sores
lodging:	sticking, attaching
longevity:	number of years to live
menstruating:	monthly bleeding cycles
midline:	middle of the body
monogamous:	sexual relations with only one partner
overtaxed:	overburdened
plague:	widespread, serious disease
precursor:	beginning
probability:	likelihood
prospective:	future
pus:	fluid from infection
shafts:	long part
spitting up:	coughing up blood
surpassed:	greater than
take hold:	become established
the like:	similar things
throw caution to the winds:	behave carelessly
upbringing:	how we were raised
vector:	insects or animals carrying diseases
verifies:	proves
weakened:	not strong
would-be:	attempted

CHAPTER 20
NONINFECTIOUS CONDITIONS: THE MODERN MALADIES

Chapter Overview

Noninfectious and chronic diseases are usually not transmitted by any pathogen or by any form of personal contact. They often develop over a long length of time, and they cause progressive damage to human tissues. Lifestyle and personal health habits are often implicated as underlying causes; however, there are a number of "newer" maladies that have unknown causes.

Chronic lung diseases pose a significant threat to Americans today. They are the fourth-leading cause of death, with most sufferers living with chronic dyspnea. Among the most deadly of the chronic lung diseases are the chronic obstructive pulmonary diseases, made up of diseases such as asthma, emphysema, and chronic bronchitis. Other respiratory ailments cause significant suffering. The most common of these are allergy-induced problems and hay fever. Allergies are a result of the body's attempt to defend itself against a specific antigen or allergen by producing specific antibodies. Hay fever attacks are characterized by sneezing and itchy, watery eyes and nose. Asthma is characterized by attacks of wheezing, difficulty in breathing, shortness of breath, and coughing spasms. Emphysema involves the gradual destruction of the alveoli of the lungs. As the alveoli are destroyed, the affected person finds it more and more difficult to exhale. In chronic bronchitis, the bronchial tubes become so inflamed and swollen that normal respiratory function is impaired. Symptoms of chronic bronchitis include a productive cough and shortness of breath that persist for several weeks. Sleep apnea is a condition of repetitive cessation of breathing during sleep.

Two forms of neurological disorders include headaches and seizure disorders. Headaches may result from dilated blood vessels within the brain, underlying organic problems, or excessive stress and anxiety. The most common forms of headaches are tension, migraine, secondary, and psychological headaches. There are several forms of seizure disorders, including grand mal, petit mal, psychomotor, and Jacksonian seizures.

Common gender-related disorders include fibrocystic breast condition, premenstrual syndrome, and endometriosis. Fibrocystic breast condition is a common noncancerous problem among women in the United States. Symptoms range in severity from a small palpable lump to large masses of irregular tissue found in both breasts. Premenstrual syndrome is a series of characteristic symptoms that occur prior to menstruation in some women. Premenstrual syndrome is characterized by depression, tension, irritability, headaches, tender breasts, bloated abdomen, backache, abdominal cramps, acne, fluid retention, diarrhea, and fatigue. Endometriosis is characterized by the abnormal growth and development of endometrial tissue in regions of the body other than the uterus. Symptoms include severe cramping during and between menstrual cycles, irregular periods, unusually heavy or light menstrual flow, abdominal bloating, fatigue, painful bowel movements with periods, painful intercourse, constipation, diarrhea, menstrual pain, infertility, and low back pain.

Digestion-related disorders include diabetes, lactose intolerance, colitis and irritable bowel syndrome, diverticulosis, peptic ulcers, and gallbladder disease. Diabetes occurs when the pancreas fails to produce enough insulin to regulate sugar metabolism or when the body fails to use insulin effectively. Diabetics exhibit hyperglycemia and high glucose levels in their urine. Other symptoms include excessive thirst, frequent urination, hunger, tendency to tire easily, wounds that heal slowly, numbness or tingling in the extremities, changes in vision, skin eruptions, and, in women, a tendency toward vaginal yeast infections. People who suffer from lactose intolerance have lost the ability to produce the digestive enzyme lactase, which is necessary for the body to convert milk sugar into glucose. Colitis is a disease of the large intestine in which the mucous membranes of the intestinal walls become inflamed. Symptoms include bloody diarrhea, severe stomach cramps, weight loss, nausea, sweating, and fever. Related to colitis is irritable bowel syndrome which is characterized by nausea, pain, gas, diarrhea attacks, or cramps after eating specific foods or when a person is under unusual stress. Diverticulosis occurs when the walls of the intestine become weakened for unknown reasons and small pea-sized bulges develop. These bulges often fill with feces and, over time, become irritated and infected. If this irritation persists, bleeding and chronic obstruction may occur, either of which can be life-threatening. Peptic ulcers occur when stomach acids irritate the stomach or intestinal lining. It is caused by the erosive effect of digestive juices on these tissues. Gallbladder disease is a result of the gallbladder being repeatedly irritated by chemicals, infection, or overuse, thus reducing its ability to release bile used for the digestion of fats. One of the characteristic symptoms of gallbladder disease is acute pain in the upper right portion of the abdomen after eating fatty foods.

Musculoskeletal diseases include arthritis, fibromyalgia, systemic lupus erythematosus (SLE), scleroderma, Raynaud's syndrome, and low back pain. Symptoms of arthritis range from the occasional tendinitis of the weekend athlete to the terrible pain of rheumatoid arthritis. Osteoarthritis is a progressive deterioration of bones and joints. Rheumatoid arthritis is an inflammatory joint disease. Symptoms may be gradually progressive or sporadic, with occasional unexplained remissions. Rheumatoid arthritis typically attacks the synovial membrane, which produces th lubricating fluids for the joints. Advanced rheumatoid arthritis often involves destruction of the bony ends of joints. Fibromyalgia is a chronic, painful rheumatological-like disorder. The cause of fibromyalgia is unknown. The disease primarily affects women in their 30s and 40s, and it causes more chronic pain and debilitation than other musculoskeletal disorders. Lupus is a disease in which the immune system attacks the body, producing antibodies tha destroy or injure organs such as the kidneys, brain, and heart. The symptoms vary from mild to severe and may disappear for periods of time. A butterfly-shaped rash covering the bridge of the nose and both cheeks is common. Nearly all SLE sufferers have aching joints and muscles, and many develop redness and swelling that moves from joint to joint. Scleroderma (hardening of the skin) is a disease characterized by an increasing fibrous growth of connective tissue underlying the skin and body organs. Scleroderma may cause swelling of the hands, face, or feet. Symptoms range from minor discomfort to severe pain. For people suffering from Raynaud's syndrome, fingers and toes may go numb, then turn white, then deep purple. As fingers and toes warm, they throb. Raynaud's is caused by exaggerated constriction of small arteries in the extremities that results in blood moving away from them and toward the vital organs. Low back pain episodes may result from muscular damage and be short-lived and acute, or may involve dislocations, fractures, or other problems with spinal vertebrae or discs and be chronic or require surgery.

Other maladies have surfaced that seem to be products of our times. Chronic fatigue syndrome and repetitive stress injuries, such as carpal tunnel syndrome, have recently received the most attention. The diagnosis of chronic fatigue syndrome depends on two major criteria and eight or more minor criteria. The major criteria are debilitating fatigue that persists for at least six months and the absence of diagnoses of other illnesses that could cause the symptoms. Minor criteria include headaches, fever, sore throat, painful lymph nodes, weakness, fatigue after exercise sleep problems, and rapid onset of these symptoms. Carpal tunnel syndrome can result in irritation to the median nerve in the wrist, causing numbness, tingling, and pain in the fingers and hands.

Learning Objectives

1. Discuss the chronic lung diseases, including allergies, hay fever, asthma, emphysema, chronic bronchitis, as well as other problems.

2. Explain the common neurological disorders, including the varied types of headaches and seizure disorders.

3. Describe the common gender disorders, risk factors for these conditions, their symptoms, and methods of their control or prevention.

4. Discuss diabetes and other digestive-related disorders, including their symptoms, prevention, and control.

5. Discuss the varied musculoskeletal diseases, including arthritis and other bone and joint problems, and their effects on the body.

6. Describe chronic fatigue syndrome and job-related disorders.

Key Terms

Fill in a brief definition to help you remember these terms.

hysterectomy ____________________

insulin ____________________

diabetes mellitus ____________________

hyperglycemia ____________________

ulcerative colitis ____________________

irritable bowel syndrome (IBS) ____________________

lactose intolerance ____________________

diverticulosis ____________________

peptic ulcer ____________________

arthritis ____________________

osteoarthritis ____________________

rheumatoid arthritis ____________________

fibromyalgia ____________________

lupus ____________________

scleroderma ____________________

Raynaud's syndrome ____________________

carpal tunnel syndrome ____________________

idiopathic ____________________

allergy ____________________

histamines ____________________

hay fever ____________________

asthma ______________________________

emphysema ______________________________

alveoli ______________________________

chronic bronchitis ______________________________

sleep apnea______________________________

migraine ______________________________

epilepsy ______________________________

fibrocystic breast condition ______________________________

premenstrual syndrome (PMS) ______________________________

endometriosis ______________________________

Short Answers

1. Describe the steps of an allergy response.

2. What is the major risk factor for chronic bronchitis?

3. What are the most common forms of seizure disorders?

4. What is fibrocystic breast condition?

5. What are the symptoms of diabetes?

6. Identify the "five f's" of risk factors for gallbladder disease.

7. Describe systemic lupus erythematosus.

8. Identify risk factors for low back pain.

Critical Thinking Exercises

Dan has a history of diabetes in his family and is concerned about his degree of risk for developing the disease. What characteristics would place Dan at greater risk for diabetes?

Gary has been diagnosed with a peptic ulcer. What should he avoid so that his condition is not exacerbated?

3. Angela has been diagnosed with chronic fatigue syndrome. What can she expect for treatment?

4. Olivia is a typist for a publishing company. She was recently diagnosed with carpal tunnel syndrome. Describe her condition, and discuss how she can alleviate her suffering.

Critical Thinking Activity: The Family and Medical Leave Act

Chronic diseases such as migraine headaches, premenstrual syndrome, and low back pain cause American workers substantial pain, suffering, and disability. Partially in response to the high incidence of chronic diseases among American workers, Congress passed the Family and Medical Leave Act (FMLA), which gives eligible employees the right to take unpaid leave, or earned paid leave, for up to 12 work weeks in any 12 months because of the birth, adoption, or foster care of a child; because the employee is needed to care for a family member with a serious health condition; or because the employee's own serious health condition makes the employee unable to do his or her job.

List the pros and cons of the FMLA. Form your own conclusion as to the merits of the FMLA, and explain your reasoning.

Language Enrichment Glossary

In addition to the words in the Key Terms list at the end of the chapter, students listed the following words as difficult to understand. Use the Key Terms list, this list, your dictionary, and teachers and friends to learn the meaning of words you do not understand.

acute: intense
allergen: substance that causes an allergic reaction
antibodies: body substance which protects against infections or allergens
antigen: substance that causes production of antibodies
bloated: swollen
bone fusion: join bones
characterized by: shown by
clamped: fastened
congenital: inborn
controversial: not commonly agreed upon
convened: gathered
correlate: associate
cramps: painful muscle contractions
criteria: measurements
debilitating: weakening
dilated: expanded
dilation/constriction: expanding/contracting
disoriented: confused, lost
dissuade: persuade not to do something
empowering: giving a sense of worth
erosive: erodes, deteriorates
etiology: origin, cause
exacerbate: make worse
excruciatingly: agonizingly, intensely
extensive: broad, thorough
functional mobility: ability to move
geared towards: directed to, focused on
generated: created
host: large number
hypersensitivity: overreaction
inadvertently: unintentionally
incidence: frequency
inflamed: irritated, red, swollen
inflammation: swelling, infection
inhalers: medical breath sprays to improve breathing
inroads: to make progress
insidious: not obvious
intractable: stubborn
irrespective: regardless
judicious: careful
lactose intolerance: inability to digest milk products
lanky: tall, thin
maladies: illnesses
nauseated: sick to the stomach

noninvasive:	not damaging
old standby:	traditional, reliable
overt:	obvious,-easy to see
overzealous:	trying too hard
particulate matter:	tiny airborne particles
plagued:	bothered by
plateaued:	leveled off
plausible:	believable
precipitating event:	cause
prognosis:	expectation of recovery
progressive damage:	worsening, spreading
pulsating:	pounding, throbbing
radiating:	spreading
rationale:	reason
regulate:	control
relapse:	occur again
remission:	disappearance
retraction:	pull back
risk factor:	associated danger, cause
scrutinize:	examine carefully
seizure:	convulsion
sporadic:	irregular, periodic
static positions:	held in one place without moving
stunning:	surprising, amazing
subjective:	opinion of the individual
substantiated by:	supported by
synthetic:	artificial substance
theorize:	propose
thrash around:	move back and forth rapidly
trivialized:	treated as unimportant
trunk:	torso, upper body
turf wars:	disagreements over responsibilities
undue:	excessive
validated:	confirmed, proved
warming up:	stretching muscles before exercise
wheezing:	breathing difficulty

CHAPTER 21
HEALTHY AGING: A LIFELONG PROCESS

Chapter Overview

Aging is defined as the patterns of life changes that occur in members of all species as they grow older. Discrimination against people based on age is known as ageism. When directed against the elderly, this type of discrimination means social ostracism and negative portrayals of older people. A developmental task approach to life-span changes tends to reduce the potential for ageism. The study of gerontology explores the reasons for aging and the ways in which people cope with and adapt to this process. Gerontologists have identified several types of age-related characteristics to determine a person's life-stage development. Biological age refers to the relative age or condition of the person's organs and body systems. Psychological age is a person's adaptive capacities, such as coping abilities and intelligence. Social age refers to a person's habits and roles relative to society's expectations. Legal age is based on chronological years and is used to determine such things as voting rights and eligibility for Social Security. Functional age is used to compare individuals of similar ages. People aged 65 to 74 are classified as young-old; those aged 75 to 84 are the middle-old group; and those 85 and over are classified as the old-old.

While the 65 and older group makes up one in 8 of all Americans today, it will include one in 6 by the year 2020. The swelling numbers of elderly will have a growing impact on our society in terms of economy, health care, housing, and ethical considerations.

Of the various theories about the biological causes of aging, the following are among the most commonly accepted: the wear-and-tear theory, the cellular theory, the autoimmune theory, and the genetic mutation theory. Numerous psychological and sociological factors also influence the aging process. The psychosocial theories of Erikson and Peck both stress the incorporation of age-related factors into lifelong behavior patterns.

As we grow older, physical changes occur in the skin, bones and joints, head features, the urinary tract, the heart and lungs, the senses, sexual function, and regulation of body temperature. Intelligence does not decline with age, although the elderly may have some problems with short-term memory. Those who have developed self-confidence, self-reliance, healthy attitudes, and effective coping mechanisms typically lead active lives in their old age. But for those who do experience mental and emotional problems, the most common are depression, senility, and Alzheimer's disease.

Health challenges of the elderly include alcohol abuse, prescription drug use and over-the-counter drug interactions, and caregiving issues. Actions for healthy aging include developing and maintaining healthy relationships, enriching the spiritual side of life, improving fitness, and eating for healthy older years.

Learning Objectives

1. Review the definition of aging, and explain the related concepts of biological age, psychological age, social age, legal age, and functional age.

2. Explain the impact on society of the growing population of the elderly, including considerations of economics, health care, living arrangements, and ethical and moral issues.

3. Discuss the biological and psychosocial theories of aging and examine how knowledge of these theories may have an impact on your own aging process.

4. Identify the major physiological changes that occur as a result of the aging process.

5. Discuss the unique health challenges faced by the elderly, such as alcohol abuse, prescription medication and over-the-counter drug use, osteoporosis, urinary incontinence, depression, senility, and Alzheimer's disease.

6. Examine the differences between males and females in terms of their numbers among the elderly population and of their roles as caregivers for others.

Key Terms

Fill in a brief definition to help you remember these terms.

aging ______________________________

ageism ______________________________

gerontology ______________________________

young-old ______________________________

middle-old ______________________________

old-old ______________________________

osteoporosis ______________________________

urinary incontinence ______________________________

cataracts ______________________________

glaucoma ______________________________

senility ______________________________

Alzheimer's disease ______________________________

comorbidity ______________________________

respite care ______________________________

sarcopenia______________________________

Short Answers

1. What is the study of gerontology?

2. What is functional age? How is this age-related characteristic assessed?

3. Distinguish between the young-old, middle-old, and old-old.

4. Profile today's elderly in terms of average life expectancy and percent of total population.

5. What are the living arrangements of the majority of the elderly?

6. How does the wear-and-tear theory explain aging?

7. What do the psychosocial theories of both Erikson and Peck stress about successful aging?

8. Identify risk factors for developing osteoporosis.

9. What physiological changes in the senses occur as a result of the aging process?

10. List three sexual changes which generally occur with aging for males and females.

11. What are the three stages of Alzheimer's disease?

Critical Thinking Exercises

1. At age 65, Sam became eligible for his Social Security benefits. This relates to which age-related characteristic?

2. As a young adult, Lisa has just learned that she is at risk for osteoporosis and is concerned about developing the disease. What steps can she take to prevent osteoporosis now?

3. Pam wonders about her grandmother's inability to remember where she went shopping yesterday, while she can clearly recall the details of when she came to Ellis Island as a child 75 years ago. Explain this phenomenon among the elderly.

4. Among the changes associated with the aging process discussed in the text, which concern you most? Why?

____

____

____

____

____

Critical Thinking Activity: An Interview on Aging

Your textbook is full of interesting information about the aging process, but no textbook can adequately describe what it is really like to grow old. You need to talk with someone who has experienced the aging process firsthand. Select someone you know who is 65 or older and with whom you can communicate openly and honestly. Ask him/her to help you complete the following critical thinking activity.

AGING QUESTIONNAIRE

Name ______________________________

Age __________

1. How has your health changed in recent years?

2. How frequently do you see your children and grandchildren?

3. Do you exercise regularly? If so, in what way?

4. What is the best thing about growing older?

5. What is most difficult about growing older?

6. What groups or activities do you enjoy that are just for older people?

7. Have you ever experienced prejudice based on your age? Explain.

8. What is the effect of the aging process on your memory?

9. What is the effect of the aging process on your intelligence?

10. How old do you *feel?*

Language Enrichment Glossary

In addition to the words in the Key Terms list at the end of the chapter, students listed the following words as difficult to understand. Use the chapter Key Terms list, this list, your dictionary, and teachers and friends to learn the meaning of words you do not understand.

ageist: prejudiced based on age
autoimmune: immune system attacking itself
bedridden: confined to bed
beset: bothered by
bizarre: extremely unusual
burden: responsibility
chronological: number of years
coexist: live together
compensating: making up for
deteriorate: break down
diminishing: decreasing
disproportionately: more than expected
dose: prescribed amount
dysfunction: unhealthy relationships
earlobes: bottom part of the ear
estrogen: a female hormone
farsightedness: inability to see close objects clearly
gerontologist: one who studies aging
immobilized: unable to move
immune system: body's protection system
inflammatory: causing swelling and irritation
laxative: something to cause bowel movements
malfunction: incorrect functioning
ostracism: isolation
overburdened: too much responsibility
pathological: seen as illness
pegged: attached
perennial: constant
portrayals: pictures, ideas
predispose: create a tendency toward
privileges: rights
regimen: diet or therapy system
sag: droop, hang down
self-reliance: depending on yourself
urinate: to pass urine
vigorous: energetic

CHAPTER 22
DYING AND DEATH: THE FINAL TRANSITION

Chapter Overview

Dying is the process of decline in body functions resulting in the death of an organism. Death can be defined as the "final cessation of the vital functions" and also refers to a state in which these functions are "incapable of being restored." The concept of brain death, defined as the irreversible cessation of all functions of the entire brain stem, has gained increasing credence. We can look at our attitudes toward death on a continuum. At one end, death is viewed as the mortal enemy of humankind. At the other end of the continuum, death is accepted and even welcomed. Most of us perceive ourselves to be in the middle of this continuum. The attitudes we develop about death are influenced by many factors.

Thanatology is the study of death and dying. Kubler-Ross identified five psychological stages that terminally ill patients often experience: denial, anger, bargaining, depression, and acceptance. However, subsequent research has shown that the experiences of persons who are dying are not that specific and vary from person to person. Social death is an irreversible situation in which a person is not treated like an active member of society. The need for social support does not diminish in the face of death, and may, in fact, increase. Bereavement is defined as the loss or deprivation experienced by a survivor when a loved one dies. Because relationships vary in type and intensity, reactions to losses also vary. When a person experiences a loss that cannot be openly acknowledged, publicly mourned, or socially supported, coping may be much more difficult. Grief work is the process of integrating the reality of the loss with everyday life and learning to feel better. When an infant or child dies, the grief may be overwhelming. Siblings of the deceased child have a particularly hard time with grief work. Social and emotional support for the bereaved in the aftermath of death is supported by many cultures. Typically, however, there is little support for many other significant losses in life. These quasi-death experiences resemble death in that they involve separation, termination, loss, and a change in identity or self-perception. If grief results from these losses, the pattern of the grief response will probably be similar to responses to death.

There are different types of terminal care available today. An increasing number of people are considering the hospice philosophy as an acceptable alternative to modern "high-tech" death. The primary goals of the hospice program are to relieve the dying person's pain, to offer emotional support to the dying person and loved ones, and to restore a sense of control to the dying person, the family, and friends. Many people prefer to go to a hospital to die. Others choose to die at home, without the intervention of medical staff or life-prolonging equipment. Each dying person and his or her family should decide as early as possible what type of terminal care is most desirable and feasible. Funerals assist survivors of the deceased in coping with their loss. Preplanning of funerary details reduces the stress on survivors and is becoming more acceptable in our culture. Decisions should be made in advance about the issue of wills and organ donation.

The right to die, rational suicide, and euthanasia are all controversial concepts in the study of death and dying. Many people today believe that they have the right to die if they have a terminal condition and their existence is dependent on mechanical life support devices or artificial feeding or hydration systems. As long as a person is conscious and competent, he or she has the legal right to refuse treatment, even if this decision will hasten death. However, when a person is in a coma or is otherwise incapable of speaking on his or her behalf, medical personnel and administrative policy will dictate treatment. The living will was developed to assist in resolving conflicts among these people and agencies. Thousands of terminally ill people decide to kill themselves rather than endure constant pain and slow decay. The issue of rational suicide involves ethical, moral, and legal issues. Dyathanasia involves someone playing a passive role in the death of a terminally ill person. The term active euthanasia means to end the life of a person who is suffering greatly and has no chance of recovery. Passive euthanasia refers to the intentional withholding of treatment that would prolong life.

Learning Objectives

1. Discuss and evaluate why people deny death.
2. Discuss the stages of the grieving process and describe several strategies for coping more effectively with death.
3. Review the decisions that are necessary when someone is dying or has died, including hospice care, funeral arrangements, wills, and organ donations.
4. Describe the ethical concerns that arise from the concepts of the right to die and rational suicide.

Key Terms

Fill in a brief definition to help you remember these terms.

dying ______________________________

death ______________________________

thanatology ______________________________

social death ______________________________

bereavement ______________________________

disenfranchised grief ______________________________

grief ______________________________

mourning ______________________________

grief work ______________________________

quasi-death experiences ______________________________

hospice ______________________________

holographic will ______________________________

testator ______________________________

intestate ______________________________

dyathanasia ______________________________

Short Answers

1. What are the criteria for brain death?

2. What is the term for the study of death and dying?

3. What is *social death*?

4. Define disenfranchised grief and provide examples of losses that may lead to such grief.

5. What is the difference between grief and mourning?

6. What are the primary goals of hospice programs?

7. What is a holographic will?

Critical Thinking Exercises

1. Your cousin has just been diagnosed with a terminal illness. She asks what stages of dying she should expect to go through. Describe Kubler-Ross's stages of dying.

2. Ellen is concerned about her husband, whose father, with whom he was very close, just died. What common grief reactions can she expect to observe in her husband?

3. Dominic and Sarah's young children are affected by the death of their grandfather. How should they talk with their children about coping with their bereavement?

4. Felicia's brother is conscious and competent, but he has several vital organs that are about to give out. The doctors plan to put him on artificial life support. Without artificial life support, he cannot survive. Can he legally refuse treatment? Why or why not?

5. Suppose your close friend has a terminal illness. Your friend raises the subject of rational suicide and wants you to explain the basic arguments for and against rational suicide. What would you say?

Critical Thinking Activity: A Look at Funeral Homes

Funeral rituals tell a lot about our culture's view of death. Collect and review written information from three funeral homes concerning services offered and costs involved. Then consider the following questions:

1. What do the materials suggest about the importance of a funeral?

2. What role does a funeral serve?

3. What does a funeral cost?

4. What are the advantages of preplanning a funeral?

5. Does it make you uncomfortable to review this information? Why or why not?

Language Enrichment Glossary

In addition to the words in the Key Terms list at the end of the chapter, students listed the following words as difficult to understand. Use the Key Terms list, this list, your dictionary, and teachers and friends to learn the meaning of words you do not understand.

actuality:	reality
alienation:	isolation
alleviation:	reduced, soothed
anticipate:	predict ahead of time
apathy:	indifferent, lack of interest
apprehension:	anxiety, worry
arduous:	hard, difficult
augmenting:	increasing, adding to
cognitive ability:	thinking ability
comprehensive:	thorough, inclusive
contemporaries:	colleagues
contend:	deal with
contestable:	opposed, debated
controversy:	disagreement
curtailed:	decreased or ended
debilitating:	weakening
designated:	specified, chosen
differentiated:	separated
dignified:	honorable, respectful
directive:	written order
disenfranchised:	to take away a right or privilege
dissident:	someone who disagrees with the majority
ecstasy:	great joy
embalmed:	treated with chemicals to preserve, slow decay
embraced:	enthusiastic agreement
equated with:	compared to
ethical dilemmas:	moral puzzles, difficulties
euphemism:	gentler word for offensive word
euthanasia:	helping one who wants to die
exile:	to be sent away from
extension:	lengthening
facilitate:	simplify, make easy
false reassurance:	untrue encouragement
fixed and dilated:	staring and expanded
fortified:	strengthened
futile:	hopeless, useless

humane:	kind, merciful
imminent:	approaching
impending:	upcoming
impersonal:	detached, impartial
in accordance with:	agrees with
indicator:	evidence, a sign
individually characteristic:	associated with one individual
insomnia:	inability to sleep
integrate:	combine, unite
interdisciplinary:	from several different specialties
intrinsic:	natural, inborn
kept under wraps:	hidden
mediated:	outsider helps to solve a problem
medical ethicists:	specialists who decide medical moral problems
nonconformists:	people who don't follow common behavior
obituary:	public death notice
paradoxical:	contradictory
pervasive:	widespread
postmortem:	after death
predominant:	significant, primary
prescribed:	assigned, established
rational:	logical, thought out
rattle on:	talk endlessly
remains problematic:	still a problem
reprieve:	delay
sanctity:	sacredness
scrupulous:	careful, painstaking, precise
sensationalized:	used to stimulate strong public curiosity
sensory input:	information perceived through the senses
shunted aside:	pushed away
stunned:	shocked
sullen:	gloomy, sulky
sustained:	experienced, been the receiver of
symbolic claims:	unreal demands
terminal:	ending, final
undue:	unnecessary, unreasonable
unerring:	perfect
validate:	confirm
vigorous:	active

CHAPTER 23
ENVIRONMENTAL HEALTH: THINKING GLOBALLY, ACTING LOCALLY

Chapter Overview

Environmental awareness has grown tremendously since the first Earth Day in April 1970. The most challenging environmental problem is population growth. World population is increasing at unprecedented rates. Population experts believe that unless current birth and death rates change radically, 10.4 billion people will be competing for the world's diminishing resources by the year 2029.

Reducing air pollution is another environmental challenge. Congress enacted the Clear Air Act Amendments of 1990 to develop standards for six of the most widespread air pollutants: sulfur dioxide, particulates, carbon monoxide, nitrogen dioxide, ozone, and lead. Photochemical smog is a brown, hazy mix of particulates and gases that forms when oxygen-containing compounds of nitrogen and hydrocarbons react in the presence of sunlight. Long-term exposure to smog produces serious health risks, particularly for children, the elderly, pregnant women, and people with chronic respiratory disorders. Acid rain is precipitation that has fallen through acidic air pollutants, particularly those containing sulfur dioxides and nitrogen dioxides. The single greatest source of acid rain in the United States is coal-fired power plants, followed by ore smelters and steel mills. The effects of acid rain include damage to lake and pond habitats; the destruction of millions of trees in forests in Europe and North America; respiratory problems; possible hazard to a pregnant woman's unborn child; metals leaching out of the soil and lakes and making their way into water or food supplies, causing cancer in humans who consume the water and food; crop damage; and the destruction of public monuments and structures. There are between 20 and 100 potentially dangerous chemical compounds in the average American home. Indoor air pollution comes primarily from six sources: woodstoves, furnaces, asbestos, passive smoke, formaldehyde, and radon. Pollution is depleting the earth's protective ozone layer. Pollution is causing a global warming trend, which adversely affects agriculture and human health. The use of renewable resources such as solar, wind, and water power as the providers of most of the world's energy, as well as shifting away from automobiles as the primary source of transportation, will reduce air pollution significantly.

There are two general types of water pollution--point source and nonpoint source. Major categories of point source pollutants are sewage treatment plants and industrial facilities. Nonpoint pollutants result from a variety of human land use practices, such as soil erosion and sedimentation, construction wastes, and sewage sludge. Most chemicals designed to dissolve grease and oil are called organic solvents. Organic solvents work their way into the water supply in different ways. After a while, the chemicals leach into the groundwater system. A related group of toxic substances contains chlorinated hydrocarbons, such as the polychlorinated biphenyls and the dioxins.

Noise pollution affects our hearing. Symptoms of noise-related distress include disturbed sleep patterns, headaches, and tension. Short-term exposure reduces productivity, concentration levels, and attention spans, and may affect mental and emotional health. Prolonged exposure to some noises results in hearing loss.

Many areas of the United States currently face serious problems in safely and effectively managing their garbage. Each day every person in the United States generates about 4 pounds of municipal solid waste. While recycling accounts for only 13 percent of garbage treatment, experts believe that as much as 90 percent of our trash is ultimately recyclable. The U.S. government established Superfund to clean up chemical dump sites that endanger public health and land. To date, 32,500 potentially hazardous waste sites have been identified across the nation.

Ionizing radiation is produced by photons having high enough energy to ionize atoms. Nonionizing radiation is produced by photons associated with lower-energy portions of the electromagnetic spectrum. The disposal and storage of radioactive wastes created by nuclear power plants and the possibility of reactor core meltdown pose serious threats to the environment.

Learning Objectives

1. Identify the problems associated with current levels of global population growth.

2. Discuss the major causes of air pollution, including photochemical smog and acid rain, and the global consequences of the accumulation of greenhouse gases and of ozone depletion.

3. Identify sources of water pollution and the specific chemical contaminants often found in water.

4. Describe the physiological consequences of noise pollution.

5. Distinguish between municipal solid waste and hazardous waste.

6. Discuss the health concerns associated with ionizing and nonionizing radiation.

Key Terms

Fill in a brief definition to help you remember these terms.

point source pollutants ______________________________

nonpoint source pollutants ______________________________

leachate ______________________________

polychloriated biphenyis (PCBs) ______________________________

dioxins ______________________________

pesticides ______________________________

municipal solid waste ______________________________

hazardous waste ______________________________

Superfund ______________________________

meltdown ______________________________

ionizing radiation ______________________________

nonionizing radiation ______________________________

radiation absorbed doses (rads) ______________________________

sulfur dioxide ______________________________

particulates ______________________________

carbon monoxide ______________________________

nitrogen dioxide ____

ozone ____

lead ____

hydrocarbons ____

photochemical smog ____

temperature inversion ____

acid rain ____

leach ____

asbestos ____

formaldehyde ____

radon ____

chlorofluorocarbons (CFCs) ____

greenhouse gases ____

Short Answers

1. What is the concept of zero population growth?

2. Identify sources of air pollution.

3. What are sources of acid rain? What are its consequences?

4. Identify six sources of indoor air pollution.

5. What is the ozone layer?

6. What are the consequences of global warming?

7. Identify and define two general sources of water pollution.

8. Distinguish between municipal solid waste and hazardous waste.

9. What are the five R's of recycling?

10. What are the top ten environmental factors linked to cancer?

Critical Thinking Exercises

1. Alexandra is concerned about exposure to formaldehyde in her home. What are the symptoms of formaldehyde exposure? What steps can she take to reduce her exposure to formaldehyde?

2. How can you reduce the possibility of ingesting lead if it does exist in your home's water system?

3. Michael and Ellen live near a subway. What symptoms of noise-related distress might they experience?

4. Suppose you are debating on the safety of nuclear power plants. Present an argument on how nuclear power plants are a threat to the environment.

5. Suppose that you are on a committee sponsoring Earth Day. What ways would you try to raise public awareness about the environment and how do you propose to try to carry this attitude over into their personal lives?

____

____

____

____

____

Critical Thinking Activity: Bringing Environmental Hazards Home

There are certain global environmental problems, and other environmental problems which are more local in nature. Working through federal, state, and especially local officials, determine the greatest single environmental hazard in your own community. Then answer the following questions:

1. What is the greatest single environmental hazard in your community? Is this hazard known in the community? If not, why not?

2. What community efforts are already underway to combat this hazard?

3. What governmental efforts are already underway to combat this hazard?

4. What would be the costs and benefits if this environmental hazard was eliminated?

Language Enrichment Glossary

In addition to the words in the Key Terms list at the end of the chapter, students listed the following words as difficult to understand. Use the chapter Key Terms list, this list, your dictionary, and teachers and friends to learn the meaning of words you do not understand.

aggravates:	makes worse
beget:	conceive
cling:	stick to
coincide:	happen at the same time
complacency:	contentment
decibel:	loudness
decommissioned:	taken out of use
degradation:	deterioration
depleting:	using up
diagnostic:	used to diagnose health problems
dire:	serious
discrete:	specific, separate
dissipate:	scatter, get rid of
emit:	send out
hinders:	slows or stops
inequitable:	unfair
leach:	soak
mutation:	change from normal
obscure:	hide, limit
outgassing:	sending off gas
precursor:	occurs before
predominant:	most frequent
probe:	investigation
proponents:	supporters
rely:	depend on
rooted:	based
seep:	leak
sifting:	moving
smelters:	metal refineries
surge:	rise

CHAPTER 24
CONSUMERISM: SELECTING HEALTH-CARE PRODUCTS AND SERVICES

Chapter Overview

Being an informed consumer will help you obtain optimal health care at an affordable cost. Perhaps the single greatest difficulty that we face as health consumers is the sheer magnitude of choices available to us. Wise consumers use every means available to them to ensure that they are acting responsibly in their own health choices. Advertising claims sometimes appear to be supported by spontaneous remission and the placebo effect.

A recent concept in health consumerism is that the patient is the primary health care provider, which means knowing your own body and its signals and taking action to stop the progression of illness or injury or to improve your overall health. Effective self-care also means knowing when you need professional medical attention. If you need medical help, you must then identify what type you need and where to obtain it. Knowledge of both allopathic medical specialties and alternative medicine and an awareness of your own criteria for evaluating a health care professional are necessary to make an informed decision. In considering prospective health care providers, you need to take into account the professional educational training they have had and if they are affiliated with an accredited medical facility or institution.

Allopathic medicine is traditional, Western medical practice. In theory, it is based on scientifically validated methods and procedures. Medical alternatives to traditional medicine are called nonallopathic medicine. Examples of nonallopathic medicine include chiropractic treatment, acupuncture, herbalists and homeopaths, and naturopathy.

There are different types of medical practices available. Physicians in group practice share the same offices, equipment, utility bills, staff costs, and profits. Solo practitioners are doctors who practice independently of other practitioners. Both hospitals and clinics provide a spectrum of health care, including emergency treatment, diagnostic tests and inpatient and outpatient care. Selection of a hospital or clinic will depend on your particular needs, income, insurance coverage, and the availability of services in your community.

Issues facing today's health care system include cost, access, quality, and malpractice. Factors that contribute to rising health-care costs include excessive administrative costs, duplication of services, and the growth of, use of, and demand for new diagnostic and treatment technologies. Your access to health care depends on the supply of providers and facilities, your health status, and your insurance coverage. The U.S. health-care system employs several mechanisms for assuring quality services overall: education, licensure, certification/registration, accreditation, peer review, and the legal system of malpractice litigation. A newer form of quality measurement uses "outcome" as the main indicator for measuring health-care quality at the individual level.

The fundamental principle of insurance underwriting is that the cost of health care can be predicted for large populations. Policyholders pay premiums into a pool, which fills as reserves until needed. When you are sick or injured, the insurance company pays out of the pool, regardless of your total amount of contribution. Unfortunately, not everyone has health insurance. Contrary to the common belief that the uninsured are unemployed, 75 percent are either workers or the dependents of workers. For the uninsured and many of the underinsured, health care may not be available through any source because of their inability to pay. Insurance is provided by private insurance companies and the government Medicare and Medicaid programs. Managed care describes a health care delivery system comprised of a budget, a network of providers, and an established set of administrative rules. Many such plans pay their contracted health care providers through capitation. Several basic models of health-care reform have been proposed.

Learning Objectives

1. Discuss the methods advertisers use to attract, switch, and maintain customers.

2. Explain when self-diagnosis and self-care are appropriate, when you should seek traditional or non-traditional health care, and how to assess health care professionals.

3. Compare and contrast allopathic and nonallopathic medicine, including the types of treatment that fall into each category.

4. Discuss the types of health care available, including types of health care practices, hospitals, and clinics.

5. Examine the current problems associated with our changing health-care system, including cost, access, choice of treatment modality and quality.

6. Describe health insurance options, including private insurance coverage, Medicare, Medicaid, and managed care choices (HMOs and PPOs).

Key Terms

Fill in a brief definition to help you remember these terms.

spontaneous remission ________________________________

placebo effect ________________________________

allopathic medicine ________________________________

primary care practitioner ________________________________

osteopath ________________________________

ophthalmologist ________________________________

optometrist ________________________________

dentist ________________________________

orthodontist ________________________________

oral surgeon ________________________________

nurse ________________________________

nonallopathic medicine ________________________________

chiropractic medicine ________________________________

group practice ________________________________

solo practitioner ______________________________

nonprofit (voluntary) hospitals ______________________________

for-profit (proprietary) hospitals ______________________________

outpatient (ambulatory) care ______________________________

Medicare ______________________________

Medicaid ______________________________

diagnosis related groups (DRGs) ______________________________

managed care ______________________________

capitatum______________________________

Short Answers

1. People often fall victim to false health claims because they mistakenly believe that a product or provider has helped them. This belief often arises from what two conditions?

2. Identify five major medical professionals who subscribe to allopathic medical procedures.

3. Distinguish between an optometrist and an ophthalmologist.

4. Identify three examples of nonallopathic alternatives.

5. What is cost-shifting?

6. What problem does our nation have concerning access to health care?

7. Distinguish between Medicare and Medicaid.

8. What are Health Maintenance Organizations (HMOs)? What concerns have been leveled against HMOs?

Critical Thinking Exercises

1. What is meant by the concept that the patient is the primary health care provider? What are the most common forms of self-care? Of these, which do you practice?

2. Suppose you have just moved to a new city and need to find a physician. What factors should you consider about a prospective health care provider?

3. Zooey has just finished her residency in internal medicine and is deciding whether to join a group practice or to go solo. What should Zooey consider in her decision?

4. How can you be proactive in your health care?

5. The text discusses several options to deal with the health care crisis. Discuss the option most appealing to you and explain why you feel this option is the best option.

Critical Thinking Activity: Selecting a Primary Care Practitioner

There are many criteria for selecting a primary care practitioner. When it comes to those criteria, all doctors are not created equal. Choose three primary care practitioners at random out of the yellow pages. Call their offices and ask for the following information:

a. professional educational training
b. licenses or board certifications held
c. affiliations with accredited medical facilities
d. years of experience
e. weekend and evening office hours

Questions for the Critical Thinker

After compiling this information, reflect on the following questions. Your thoughtful responses will help you in the understanding of consumerism.

1. Have you ever asked these sorts of questions before? If not, why not?

2. Was it difficult to ask these questions? Why or why not?

3. How eager were the offices to answer your questions? Do you think that other consumers ask such questions in their search for a primary care practitioner?

4. What conclusions would you make about choice of primary care practitioner based on the information you received?

5. What other questions or concerns do you have about a primary care practitioner?

Language Enrichment Glossary

In addition to the words in the Key Terms list at the end of the chapter, students listed the following words as difficult to understand. Use the Key Terms list, this list, your dictionary, and teachers and friends to learn the meaning of words you do not understand.

access: admission
adamantly: in a determined manner
adverse: negative, harmful
amend: alter
arsenal: storehouse, stockpile
attribute: characteristic
catastrophic: unexpected, devastating
charlatans: fakes, impostors
condescending: done with a superior manner
consensus process: decision process in which all attempt to agree
dilemma: problem, puzzle
divert: turn aside
drastic: extreme
dubious: doubtful, untrustworthy
evolve: develop
experiential background: experience
federalization: national government supervision
fluoridation: chemicals added to public water supplies to reduce tooth decay
fraud: deceit, cheating
freestanding: existing alone
generic names: general names for a category of things
gimmicks: tricks
glaring: obvious
ground swell: public opinion
hangs tenuously: connected loosely and about to fall
HMO: health maintenance organization
humanitarian: volunteer social assistance
hypothetical: imaginary
imperative: essential, necessary
in flux: changing
incremental: small step by step
indigent: poor, without resources
infinite: endless
intimidated: scared
lobbying efforts: persuasive efforts
mandated: ordered
markedly: significantly
maze: confusing puzzle
means: methods, resources
multifactorial: including many reasons
primary care physician: general care doctor
proactive: initiate activity

prohibited:	prevented
prospective:	expected
sheer magnitude:	large size
streamlining:	simplifying
substantiated:	proved
trendy:	popular, stylish
utilization review:	review of use of services
viable options:	workable choices
warrant:	require

NOTES

NOTES

NOTES

NOTES

NOTES

NOTES

NOTES

NOTES

NOTES

NOTES